Sugar Detox

The ultimate step-by-step guide on quitting sugar and completely stop craving

Medical Disclaimer

All the material in this eBook has been carefully researched, using combinations of books, health blogs, online video, and hospital and doctor websites.

However, we must make this disclaimer:

The content and information provided in this eBook, was constructed for educational purposes only.

Regarding natural health solutions such as the Sugar Detox, the information should never be used as a substitute for medical care.

The statements regarding health-related benefits of certain ingredients may not been evaluated by the Food and Drug Administration and are in no way intended and should not be construed as medical advice to diagnose, treat, cure, or prevent any disease or health condition. As such it is not intended for you to disregard professional medical advice or delay in seeking medical attention.

The information which has been researched diligently and is never meant to substitute the advice provided by your personal physician or other medical professionals.

Please read the eBook carefully and take note of all the ingredients listed. If you are allergic or sensitive to any of the ingredients, which may be contained in the products, natural food or drink, ask your doctor of any possible short or long term affects. Even natural ingredients may cause sensitivities. Each person is different, and since you may or may not have ingested a particular food or drink, we cannot guarantee you will not get a reaction or irritation.

People with severe allergies should be diligent. If you have severe anaphylactic-type reactions to any of the ingredients, do not consume them.

The authors of this material are not liable for any medical situations that may arise, as the disclaimer clearly states caution and self-responsibility.

Table Of Content

Introduction

- Why Is Sugar Bad for You? 6
- Health Problems Caused By Sugar.................................... 7
- The Negative Impact of Sugar on the Brain................ 8
- The Negative Effects Of Sugar On Skin......................... 9
- The Health Benefits of a Sugar Detox......................... 10
- What Happens When You Stop Eating Sugar? 11
- The Science Behind Sugar Cravings.............................12

The 4-Week Plan For Your Sugar Detox

- Getting Ready Before The Detox Starts......................15
- Week #1.. 20
- Week #2.. 26
- Week #3.. 29
- Week #4.. 31

Practical Fast Track Guides and Listings

- Yes/No Foods... 33
- Guide To Hidden Sugars... 38
- Sugar Detox Shopping List... 39
- Understanding Ingredients On Food Labels............... 40
- Guide To Dining Out.. 42

Starter Recipes For Your Three Main Meals

- 7 Breakfast Recipes.. 44

- 7 Lunch Recipes.. 49
- 7 Main Dishes Recipes... 56
- 7 Recipes to Replace Traditional Desserts.................. 64
- 7 Snacks & Sides Recipes.. 74

Conclusion... or not?

Introduction

Why Is Sugar Bad for You?

Out of all the things we ingest, sugar is the one that can do the most damage. It has been proven to have a negative effect on us, physically and mentally. There are different types of sugars that are currently in the average person's diet.

We see refined white sugar, brown sugar, corn fructose in a wide variety of products. Even too much natural sugars from fruits can have negative effect on our blood sugars.

A diet high in sugar can lead to diabetes, heart issues and decreased brain function. High sugar diets means that people are likely ingesting foods like donuts, cake and pop. This contributes to bad fats in the blood stream and the liver.

Studies have shown that cancer likes to feed off the sugar in our bodies. By having a high sugar diet, it is encouraging the body to get sick instead being healthy.

Health Problems Caused By Sugar

Most people understand that eating a diet high in sugar, normally results in obesity. Studies have been done on sugar consumption throughout the world and the United States leads in this unwanted record. Consumption of fast food due to the proliferation of restaurants pumping out fast sugar laden foods is one of the leading causes. Advertising is huge in the United States and companies spend millions to get consumers hooked on their products. Eating a diet based on high sugar content, can be destructive to your health.

We are all aware that sugar causes tooth decay. What may not be totally explained by the dentist, is the fact that it also contributes to gum disease. Thinking about having gum disease may cause some unpleasant internal pictures in the mind, yet the worst is yet to come. Chronic gum disease can cause heart disease by having an impact on the arteries of the heart.

While the immune system is a hot topic due to colds, the flu and other viruses, it should be known that sugar causes the immune system to malfunction. Bacteria and cells prone to cancer, feed off sugar and grow. Without a healthy immune system to keep things in check, it can lead to serious health issues.

The Negative Impact of Sugar on the Brain

Our body is made of cells that require fuel to survive. Studies have shown that we use only a small portion of our brain, unless we make it a priority to work on upping our brain's capacity for work.

The brain contains the majority of the nerves in the body and those nerves require glucose to function. When you are addicted to sugar, it is possible you are ingesting as much as 2 to 3 times the daily recommended amount.

When this occurs, it alters the mood drastically. There is likely to be an increase in depression and anxiety.

Researchers have found that diets high in sugar, react similarly when cocaine is introduced to the body. Scans show certain nerves firing up with sugar or cocaine ingested, which is why so many people feel addicted to the need for sugar.

Proper insulin production is needed to maintain blood sugar levels. Unfortunately, sugar impedes on the insulin in your body and makes it less effective. The balanced insulin works to keep your brain health functioning properly and when the insulin is not regulated, it can cause cognitive issues in the brain. This research has been backed up using the data from those who suffer from type 2 diabetes. Those who suffer from this disease have a much higher chance of developing dementia in their later years.

The Negative Effects Of Sugar On Skin

Acne can be a serious concern and it doesn't just happen to teenagers. One cause of acne breakout can be attributed to a diet high in sugar. When a person eats too much sugar, it first has an impact on their insulin levels, which then contributes to inflammation in the body. Inflammation can be found anywhere, from the muscles to even the brain. As inflammation occurs, it may happen in the facial region and this can induce an acne outbreak.

Many people are concerned with wrinkles. This will occur naturally as we age, yet sugar has been shown to increase the amount of wrinkles even at an earlier age. High amounts of sugar work against the natural collagen in the facial muscles. Collagen helps keep the skin tight and when it weakens, it does not have the ability to hold the skin properly and sagging occurs.

The Health Benefits of a Sugar Detox

There are so many benefits to doing a sugar detox and eliminating it from your diet. The reduced risk of serious disease should be very motivating. For many people, struggling with their weight causes not only health issues but emotional ones as well. Getting off sugar is number one in reducing weight. As the pounds come off and stay off, a positive mindset is much easier to keep. This means reduced stress and depression. Plus many overweight people have anxiety issues when it comes to family, friends and just being observed by strangers as they go about their daily lives.

Everyone wants to have the energy to do the things they love. They also need energy to have a successful career. By going on a sugar detox, everyone, including the people struggling with weight issues, will see a positive impact on their energy levels.

Many digestive issues are often attributed to a high consumption of sugar. As sugar is replaced by healthy vegetables, healthy fats and proteins, the issues of bloating, upset stomach and those gas attacks...will decrease dramatically.

What happens when you stop eating sugar?

Detoxing from any substance will cause some issues. This is where you have to be strong and use some grit to power through the obstacles.

You will likely have some minor headaches over the first few days. You won't be the only one, because even people who quit drinking coffee go through the same thing. The other thing you will notice is that your energy levels will drop off. With this in mind, you should probably consider scheduling your detox to start, when you are not on a mind boggling schedule, like exams or a huge project at work.

Some people report digestive issues as well. It is important that you really up the amount of water that you drink. This will help in flushing the system and drinking plenty of water helps with food cravings as your stomach will feel full.

The first two weeks is where you really need the will power to get this done. Heading into the next stretch, any minor headaches or stomach issues should disappear. You may still crave the sugar however, so keep the water intake going.

As you go through the final phase of detoxing from sugar, the cravings should be quite low.

Monitoring your weight will likely show a few pounds lost and your energy levels on the rise.

The Science Behind Sugar Cravings

The brain is a tricky little mass of nerves and other components. For example in the brain, we have the hippocampus. This has a lot of different tasks and it is the reward seeker. When you come home after a hard day at work and get a little mental message saying you deserve a reward, well that is your hippocampus speaking. As it deals with your memories, it can invoke an image and desire for a few chocolate chip cookies.

Conditioning happens because of the caudate nucleus in the brain. It stores memory and sparks behavior without you even being aware of it. You can now take notice if, the moment you wake up, or walk into the kitchen, there is an extreme desire for sugared cereal or perhaps chocolate covered donuts. Your eating habits come from this section of the brain, which means that you will need to retrain it. You can do this with determined focused effort.

Brain chemicals play a large part in sugar addiction. Medical research has shown that people who are low in serotonin suffer from anxiety, depression and even chronic obsessive compulsive disorder. They often have great difficulty in sleeping, partly from lack of serotonin and partly from obsessive worry that keeps their heart rate and blood pressure up.

With low serotonin levels, a person will seek alternate ways to make themselves feel pleasure even if it is only for a short time. How powerful is sugar? Scientists have found that sugar activates the same part of the brain that hard core drugs such as cocaine and heroin do. In fact, the studies have shown that people who are trying desperately to kick the heroin habit, will have massive sugar cravings.

The other natural drug in the brain that has to be considered, is dopamine. This drug is called the happy drug and it gets flooded through the body, when you watch a funny movie, ski down a steep hill or play any type of games with friends and family that you love.

Low dopamine in the brain, leads to boredom. Life seems empty and it is wake up, go to work, come home and eat while watching the television. After this non-exciting day, it off to bed and wake up for more of the same. The person isn't depressed, they are just going through the motions of life.

When you have a sugar addiction, you need to carefully document how you feel every day. This will lead you to discover if you are insufficient in serotonin or dopamine. Naturally bringing those brain chemicals up, will help to cure your sugar addiction. As we go through week by week and what to expect, there will be examples of how to up your brain chemicals naturally.

The 4-Week Sugar Detox Plan

Getting Ready To Start Your Sugar Detox

Before we get into what you need to do each week and what to expect, there is some preparation work. Trust that it will be worth it, to be on top of your game.

Detoxing from sugar may have side effects that are annoying. It is different with each person and we will discuss that more in a moment. The first task you need to accomplish is talking to all those who are in daily contact with you.

That means family, friends and if you work outside the home, your co-workers. Be honest and tell them that for the sake of your health, you are doing a sugar detox for a month. They need to be aware that you might be a little grouchy, have a headache or other issues. It is also important that they refrain from trying to tempt you with sweet treats or goad you into giving up before you even start.

Now be totally clear and honest with yourself. You are giving up processed sugars, those that you add to your food, or that companies fill their products with. Natural sugars occur in vegetables and fruits which you need. Those fruits and vegetables contain so many nutrients that are key to your survival.

You have probably heard of decluttering. This refers to getting rid of unwanted items in your home, office and computer. However it also refers to the garbage in your mind.

About 3 days out from starting your sugar detox, your first step is cut your sugar intake by half. That means, two creams in your coffee becomes one. Decide what you can do to make your sugar level intakes go down. The next day, cut it down again, so that the day before you begin, there is not a lot of sugar in your system and your body is starting to work on detoxing.

Now it is time to give away or throw out the sugar items in your house. Your neighbor might appreciate that unopened box of chocolate chip cookies or large unopened bottle of soda pop. Yes, it will hurt as you say goodbye to your old sugary friends. You will moving through the 4 weeks gradually. This means you won't be stopping sugar cold in the first week...instead you will eat normally, minus the junk food. Ask anyone who has tried to quit smoking, how easy it is to just stop suddenly. For this to work, you need to ease into it.

Detoxing sugar is done for health reasons and you may have multiple issues that you want to take care of. It is time to get your selfie game on. You want to snap a photo and document your torso, so you can compare at the end. If you have been troubled by skin issues, then for sure, take a snapshot of your face, and expect to see a big difference at the end.

We already said this was going to take work and one way you can make it fun and rewarding, is to start a sugar detox journal. If you aren't already doing gratitude journals and the like, now would be a good time to get on the right path.

In your journal, you want to write down everything that comes to your mind daily, as you detox. How do you feel? If you are losing motivation, tell yourself why you really want to do this. Write down what you notice about the changes in your physical body and your mental attitude. If you see a problem, address how you will tackle it. It is perfectly fine to use motivational quotes that you find in books and the internet. Anything that helps you, goes into the journal

It is time to shop. In this eBook, you will find recommended foods and recipe examples for each day. In fact, this eBook covers, breakfast, lunch, dinner, desert and snacks. We have your back on this.

While you are shopping, you should pick up a large office type calendar that you can write out your goals for the day. What will the exercise be today? How much water will you drink? (This is important because many people do not get enough water. You may find that you need to work on water consumption.)

What will be your meal today? What day of the week will you go back to the grocery store and replenish your pantry? Did you eat eggplant for the first time, like recommended in the further chapter and find it not to your taste? Write down some substitutes. Anything that can help you in your sugar detox gets written down.

Now if you are also doing this to lose weight, here is a tip. Write down your beginning weight on the 1st day. Do not weigh yourself until the end of week 2, week 3 and week 4. Everyone loses weight at a different pace.

Imagine your mindset if the first 3 to 4 days, you didn't even lose an ounce. You would likely want to give up. You will lose weight but at the end of week 2, if your weight loss just isn't happening, sit down and figure out what needs adjusting. It may be more water and more exercise because you didn't really think it was that important.

You can do this. Let's get started.

Week #1:

To begin your week, focus on staying off the junk foods, like chips and pop. Eat your normal foods. For example if a tuna fish sandwich is a normal lunch and meatloaf with potatoes is dinner, go ahead and have it.

You will drink at least two litres of water per day. Go online and check for water consumption for your size. If you weight 150 lbs, you don't need the same amount of water as someone who weighs 225 lbs.

You can start here:

https://www.slenderkitchen.com/article/how-to-calculate-how-much-water-you-should-drink-a-day

You need 7 servings of fruit and vegetables. So if you have toast in the morning, have an apple too.

Your body needs the omega 3 foods. Make sure you eat at least one serving, such as fish or avocado. This will assist your brain and help with inflammation in the body.

At some point during the week, you need to replace one meal with a bone broth. This will help with weight loss and digestive issues. Make your own bone broth, do not buy the powdered variety. Simple bone broth recipes are easy to find on the internet. If you have a freezer, make plenty and keep it on hand. Should you get a cold or flu, drink plenty of bone broth as you will not eat properly and it will help in recovery.

Everyone should be exercising, not just those on the sugar detox. For success purposes, you need to include a high intensity workout. This could be bike riding for example. Do this work out the day you replaced a meal with bone broth and do it just before your next real meal.

Check out this exercises for examples:

https://www.shape.com/fitness/workouts/hiit-workout-exercises

As you need to work on the chemical productions in your brain, let's start with serotonin. You should have decided if the issues you face are a lack of serotonin, resulting in anxiety, depression or something else. When you decide you need dopamine, then you need an action plan to get out of boredom. There will be cases where some people need both, so again putting together an action plan is essential.

Serotonin Fixers:

- Get a proper amount of safe sunlight
- Go to bed early and meditate briefly before sleeping 7-8 hours
- Relax and breathe. Do this with yoga for an example and then have a hot bath afterwards.
- When a sugar craving hits, pop a handful of berries and let them linger in your mouth. Get all the pleasurable sensation of slowly chewing them and releasing the natural sugars. During the 4 weeks, use as many serotonin foods as you can in your meal plan. Have those seeds, nuts, and delicious vegetables.
- Talk to your doctor about vitamins and herbs that are safe for you to use to increase serotonin.
- Get a massage two to three times a week
- Work on mood enhancers, such as visualizing a happy life, creating a vision board and role playing in the mirror. Role playing in the mirror, means that before you shower, you smile in the mirror while clapping your hands and doing a little wiggle. As your mood gets happy, hop in the shower and use a special sponge to really soap up in the warm water and self-massage any aching joints or muscles.

You are going to engage in something, you may have never tried before. It is time to alter your beliefs and thoughts about who you are and what you can accomplish.

To help you detox from sugar, you can try subliminal mp3's. These mp3's are usually music with hidden words of encouragement beneath the music or crashing waves.

Note: You cannot drive while listening to this. They must be done in the comfort of your home. They are safe to use, however if you have been treated or diagnosed with a serious mental health issue, please consult your doctor before using.

Here is an example you can look at:

https://www.mindmotivations.com/shop/hypnosis-sugar-addiction-mp3

Practise daily affirmations, to change how you feel about yourself. You deserve the best in life and you need to take full responsibility and make the necessary changes to be happy and successful. These are to help you boost your serotonin.

Dopamine Fixers:

In the 7 recipes each for breakfast, lunch and dinner, you will find many examples of dopamine foods to eat.

- Sardines
- Lean Beef
- Bell peppers
- Spinach
- Garlic
- Bananas
- Lemons

These are just a small example of what will help you in getting the brain boosters that you need.

Other ways to boost dopamine are to do one of the following each day:

- Go dancing
- Get funky with nail polish
- Get busy with weightlifting, martial arts, squash, tennis, hiking and birdwatching
- Join a meetup group in your interest category
- Play games with friends that require lots of interaction, like board games
- Read a ghost story for the first time in your life

- If you have a significant other, do a dress up and let's Netflix and chill. Wink, wink!
- Play with your pet or go to the local adoption center and spend time with a dog or cat.
- Learn how to throw knifes
- Try flying kites for the first time.

The list is endless, but you probably get the idea.

Things To Expect:

- A drop in energy
- Possible headaches from withdrawal
- Loss of focus, temporally
- Possible gas, bloating or diarrhea
-

Remember, everyone is different, you may experience one or all of these. It will pass quickly.

Week #2:

This week is your first assessment. Ask yourself some questions and write in your journal how you are doing. Did you run out of any foods that you need to replace and what day will you pick them up?

After self-assessment, decide if you need to stick with your normal foods as mentioned in week 1. If the answer is that you are not really finding any issues physically, make the decision if you want to bump up to eating from the meal plan described in the section: **"Starter Recipes For Your Three Main Meals."**

It would be best if you only did this 2-3 times in week 2 and for the other days, stick to your normal meals.

This week you will again eat at least 7 servings of your best vegetables and fruits. This may sound like an easy thing but as we have said many times, everyone is different. There are people who do not eat fruit or vegetables.

One example is a former salesman, now retired. This gentleman reported only eating barbequed chicken and baked potatoes, with lots of pop. No fruit and no vegetables and certainly no water. That won't be you, as you have made the decision to get healthy.

- This week you need to pick two activities that will boost your serotonin, dopamine or both.
- You will be eating one omega 3 food each day for 7 days
- Time to get down to work. Pick two meals this week that you are going to skip the food and drink bone broth. It's been said that you can skip the meal altogether and not have bone broth but frankly, the benefits of bone broth are just too good to skip.
- Like week 1, you need to do a high intensity workout before the next meal. If you didn't like any of the intensity workouts, from the link provided in week 1, please don't skip this and find one you love.
- Keep working on your journal and your positive mental outlook with the subliminals and/or positive affirmations.
- You should see less physical symptoms this week. If not and you are concerned, no harm in checking in with your doctor, to see if there is an undiagnosed issue...perhaps in your digestive system.

Things to Expect:

- The vast majority of people will find their normal energy levels are back to normal. The brain will still be sending out sugar craving signals, without much of the withdrawal symptoms. It will take time to get over the feeling that a coffee with two creams and two sugary donuts are not your go to breakfast on the fast commute to work. Work on keeping your stomach full with healthy fats and proteins, to keep the residual cravings at bay. Double check to make sure you are drinking the right amount of water. Are you keeping notes in your journal to make sure you didn't fall off the horse?

Week #3:

This week, you start dropping the huge bowl of spaghetti for dinner or that triple decker deli meat sandwich for lunch. You want to have a "normal meal," once a day in a small portion around 250 to 300 calories. Start working the meal plans provided in the meal planner section provided.

- This week you up the serotonin/dopamine activities to 3 new ones. Please pick new activities, as you need the major excitement to get those chemicals doing their jobs.
- We bump our planned missed meal to 3 this week. Switch your bone broth around from beef to chicken and for one of them, you could do a vegetable broth if you are getting bored with the others.
- Time for a high intensity workout after the missed meal and do it just before the next one you eat.
- Continue with at least one omega 3 food per day this week.
- Try switching up your chosen vegetables and fruits and get 7 of these eaten. Switching keeps you from getting bored and you discover that you actually like Brussel sprouts with salt/pepper and a splash of balsamic vinegar.

Things to Expect:

- You have likely lost some weight and your skin is starting to improve.
- The sugar cravings have died down considerably.
- Your bowel eliminations are much more regular and it is easy to go, since you are eating more fruit and drinking plenty of water.
- Many people report that they can taste food better. Their tongues perk up when they pop a raspberry into their mouth and it tastes like a bit of heaven.
- Falling off the wagon, you might have a bottle of pop and not be able to finish it because it is just too sweet.

Week #4

We are on the home stretch now. Congratulations on getting it done.

This week you will only have a "normal meal," once. Think of it as your reward for a job well done. Again it needs to be only 250 to 300 calories, so choose wisely.

- Keeping working on 7 servings of vegetables and fruits.

- This is a big week, because you will skip 4 meals. Space it out so that Mon/Wed/Fri, you are eating 3 meals a day and use the other four days for a planned skipped meal. Again it is bone broth or vegetable broth for the skipped meal.

- This week you do a high intensity workout for the 3 days, you skipped that meal. Do it just before you eat.

- Eat one serving or more if you can, of omega 3 food. This means perhaps sardines at lunch and mackerel at dinner as an example.

- We now go to 4 activities per day, to boost your serotonin and dopamine levels. Remember there

are many of these activities that can be done in a
few minutes. How about one round of darts, while
blindfolded. Just make sure you have a spotter. :)

Things to expect:

- You are looking fit and feel your energy is better
than ever.
- The sugar cravings seem like a distant memory.
Now when you want something sweet and tart,
you have a green apple dipped in cinnamon.
- You are not out of the woods, backsliding can still
occur. If chocolate bar cravings pop up, look at see
what the cause can be. Did you stop working on
your journal and your mindset? Don't be hard on
yourself, just observe and make the necessary
adjustments.

Practical Fast Track Guides and Listings

Yes / No Foods

Deciding what to eat during a sugar detox doesn't have to be hard. In fact, once you have a list of foods to eat and foods to avoid, then it is time to clean out the pantry and restock it.

Once that is done, you set up your meal plans and get cracking on new recipes to help you kick the sugar habit, lose weight and feel great.

Remember some of the foods like tomatoes and berries will have small amounts of natural sugar, so you need to eat accordingly.

Let's start with a list of foods you can eat:

1. You will be able to enjoy fresh meats such as, beef, pork chicken, turkey and fish. Try to limit the amount of beef and pork you eat and for all your meats, if you can do it, use organic.
2. Green vegetables are your go to food and they combine well with

the fresh meats and fish
mentioned above.

3.   Eggs make a great breakfast or snack.

4.   Cheese in moderation, as long as it is not processed.

5.   Avocado is delightful in many ways.

6.   Go for the green beans and change it up with the yellow. Both are tasty.

7.   Kale and spinach. Both greens are awesome. Try dicing them fine and mixing them together.

8.   Tomato. Remember there are many different types, so try them all and you won't be get bored. There is about 2 grams of natural sugar in a half cup, so don't overdo them.

9.   Radish has a very different taste, so this may even be helpful in keeping your taste buds entertained.

10.   Yum! Cheese. It is not just for mice. A one ounce serving of cheddar cheese has approximately 0.1 grams of sugar. If you ever plan to do the Keto diet, you will see cheese on the menu. Again, always

read the packaging to make sure
the sugar levels are extremely low
and eat moderately.

11.   Cucumber is a great snack. Just
       wash and scrub your cukes, then
       eat it with the rind on. You will get
       the fiber and other goodies with it.

12.   Broccoli is amazing and if you eat it
       raw, the crunch is very satisfying.
       Think of it like this. You like chips
       for the taste and the crunch. Why
       not crunch into something good
       for you.

13.   Eggplant can be eaten in different
       ways. Try roasting it as a side dish
       to go with your skinless chicken
       breast.

14.   Peppers can be used in salads,
       sliced and dipped in virgin olive oil
       for an after dinner snack.

15.   Want something to go with that
       steak? Then break out the
       asparagus. They pair up beautiful.

16.   Berries can be very helpful with a
       sugar detox. Choose berries that
       are very low in sugar content, like
       strawberries.

17.   Bone broth or vegetable broth is a
       huge part of the sugar detox and
       even once you are done with the

detox, keep going with the bone broth. Check out how to make bone broth here:

https://wholefully.com/bone-broth/

We just covered the main foods you can eat and there are more. For now, let's just talk about condiments because many people need something on their beef or chicken. For a sugar detox purpose, make sure you have mustard, virgin olive oil, pure avocado oil and salsa. For the salsa you need to check the brand, because only a few have very low amounts of sugar. Salsa goes well with chicken or even on a salad.

For beverages, stick with water and different types of tea.

Now for the list of foods you want to stay away from...

Note: You are going to gradually detox from some of these foods like pasta and bread, as noted in the 4 week plan.

1. Stay away from all fast foods, including subs, because you do not want to eat bread and processed meats.

2.   No snacking on crackers, give them to your parrot.
3.   Having cereal for breakfast is out.
4.   This may be tough but you need to stop eating pasta eventually.
5.   Bagels have become very popular over the years but sadly, you want to stay away from them.
6.   While we mention bagels, we cannot forget bread is off the table. Actually bread is one of the main reasons for obesity, if eaten by itself or with spreads.
7.   Gluten has become a serious health issue for many people. For the detox, any wheat or similar products containing gluten must be avoided.
8.   Alcohol is dropped from the weekly "must buy," list.
9.   Try to avoid black coffee and go for the green tea instead. Of course any coffee with cream, is definitely a big no.
10.   Another big fad is energy drinks. It doesn't matter if it is one of those big cans or those thimble sized stay awake energy drinks...you need to drop them.
11.   No more cans of pop in your fridge.
12.   Processed deli meats and canned meats are out.
13.   Don't put margarine or simulated butter on your shopping list.

Guide To Hidden Sugars

People say that English is one of the harder languages to learn. We have words like, "there and their," which really confuse anyone attempting to pick the language. Now you need to understand that food companies like to play with words. When you pick up a product and it reads, "No added sugar, or something like zero grams of sugar added," this doesn't mean it is sugar free. It just means it likely contains certain amounts of sugar and the company hopes you buy it as a sugar free product.

Speaking of language, there are a number of indigenous groups of people who have multiple words for snow. In fact one group may have as many as 53 words, describing snow.

Sugar is like that as well. We call it by many names and it is important to look at labels and know what type of sugar it contains.
Here a just a few to steer clear of:
1.	Corn syrup
2.	Dextrose
3.	Vegetable glycerin
4.	Maltose
5.	Fruit juice concentrate

Sugar Detox Shopping List

In the section called, "Foods You Can Eat," we went over the main staples. As you make your grocery list, you can add those items and what is listed below. This will give you a great start on your detox.

Make sure to have these herbs and spices. Try to grow some of them at home, so you don't run out.

Chili Powder
Basil (fresh)
Black Pepper
Brewer's Yeast
Cayenne
Chili Powder
Chipotle Powder
Chives
Cilantro
Cinnamon
Coriander
Cumin
Fennel Seeds (ground)
Garlic bundles
Ginger root
Nutmeg
Oregano
Paprika
Red Chili Flakes

Rosemary

Sage leaves
Sea Salt
Smoked Paprika
Turmeric
Unsweetened Cocoa Powder
Coconut Oil
Pure Virgin Olive Oil
Sesame Seed Oil
Unsalted Butter
Coconut Milk
Olives
Almonds
Pumpkin Seeds
Sesame Seeds
Walnuts
Fish Sauce
Hot Sauce-Use a sugar free hot like Simple Girl or
Marie Sharp's Hot Habanero
Brussel sprouts

Understanding Ingredients on Food Labels

We know that there are good fats and of course
bad fats. It is essential to learn the technical
sounding name of the bad fats, to avoid buying
those products. Consuming trans fats are bad for
your heart and overall health. When looking at

labels, check for hydrogenated fats or partially hydrogenated fats. You do not want to purchase products with that in the guide list.

Content guide lists are supposed to protect the consumer, however companies will look for ways to get around telling the consumer the truth, for fear they will not buy.

When it comes to sugar, you need to look for terms like, dehydrated cane juice, high fructose corn syrup or maltodextrin. There are many others to be concerned about, so it may even be wise to write out a list of what to avoid, until you get it memorized.

Sodium can raise the blood pressure, which in turn can cause heart problems or even a stroke. Canned legumes, beans and vegetables may be in a sodium based juice to keep them moist. If you do consume a can of kidney beans or the like, pour the can into a strainer first and completely rinse them off, to help get rid of the majority of the juice.

Buying packaged deli meats like salami or pepperoni means you will find sodium nitrates on the label. These products should not be part of your diet and when buying any product, check for nitrates, sodium benzoate, MSG or disodium. MSG or monosodium glutamate is added to products.

Health coconscious consumers will likely notice when dining out, that the menu will post, "No MSG added," because it has developed such a bad reputation.

Guide To Dining Out

You can still enjoy dining out at a real restaurant by taking a few special steps.

1. Know the restaurant first by checking it out online. See if they mention anything special, like gluten free, no MSG added or Keto friendly. This will give you a head start on what you can order.
2. Before ordering, have a good look at the menu and then ask questions. Your server may not have the answer but if you are polite and tell them you need assistance, they will get the help you need. Primarily, you need to find out if there are hidden ingredients that may have sugar. For example if you are having a beef dish, find if there is a coating, or even bread crumbs.
3. Call ahead if you want to eat a nice salad and find out what condiments they have, that are sugar free. You may need to consider bringing a small bottle of your

own balsamic vinegar or sugar free hot sauce.
4. Don't be afraid to ask for something different as a side dish. If you are having a nice piece of fish and it comes with rice, ask for a green salad.
5. The key is to be prepared, so calling ahead, researching the menu online will be of great help. Certainly you want a beverage with your meal, so it is nice to know they have a great brand of sparkling water or a selection of tea.

Starter Recipes For Your Three Main Meals

To help you get started on your Sugar Detox journey, let's look at recipes for your main meals, snacks and desserts.

7 Breakfast Recipes

A) 3 in 1 Oatmeal

Directions: Use one cup of steel cut oats, 1 cup of diced mushrooms, 1 very small diced onion and ¾ cup of your own chicken stock. This is done on the stove in a small skillet. Use 1 teaspoon of virgin olive oil and once that is heated, put in your diced onions and cook until they are clear. Add in the diced mushrooms and one teaspoon of dry thyme. When the mushrooms are cooked, stir in the one cup of steel oats and the ¾ cup of chicken stock. As oatmeal is very absorbent, you will need to add approximately one cup of water. Using a wooden spoon, stir constantly for approximately six to nine minutes. Once you have placed the oatmeal in your bowl, then add ¼ cup of walnuts or hazelnuts and stir thoroughly.

B) Mushroom, Spinach and Egg

Directions: Heat your virgin olive oil in the frying pan. Add in one small diced onion or 3 green onions chopped. Stir fry your chopped mushrooms and when they are close to being cooked, add in one cup of spinach. Keep stirring the mixture until the spinach is soft. Have 4 cracked eggs ready in a bowl and stir this mixture in. Once all is cooked, you can add sugar free hot sauce or sprinkle with smoked paprika.

C) Let's Do Mexico

Directions: You will need one package of tortilla wraps or any type of wrap that is sugar free, such as a spinach wrap. Have your tomatoes, red chillies and fresh coriander leaves on hand.

To start, finely dice up four tomatoes, one to two red chillies depending on your heat preference and two coriander leaves. Place in a bowl and stir. You can add black pepper to taste if you wish. Stir in two tablespoons of virgin olive oil.

Dice up two more coriander leaves and place them in a small mixing bowl before adding six to eight cracked eggs, depending on how many will be eating breakfast. Add virgin olive oil to the frying pan, with one teaspoon of garlic. Once the garlic is cooked, stir in the egg mixture and cook until eggs still show a bit of moisture. This tastes better than overcooked eggs.

Heat up your wraps approximately 30 seconds in the microwave and once ready, spoon the eggs along the left hand side. Then spoon some of your home made salsa alongside the eggs and roll once, then close the ends and complete your rolling.

D) Peanut Butter and Banana Breakfast Smoothie

Directions:
You want amazing taste, you got it. The trick with this smoothie is finding unsweetened almond milk. You may have to research a few stores online before finding the right product.

To put it together, grab your blender and add in one banana, one tablespoon of organic peanut butter and ½ cup of that unsweetened almond milk. You want this drink to be cold, so have three to four ice cubes on the ready, to put in and blend until thoroughly mixed.

E) Powerhouse Green Breakfast Smoothie

Directions: This smoothie is not only sugar free, it is also gluten free. You need:
- One green apple diced so your blender isn't overworked.

- A cup of spinach or kale, wash thoroughly.
- One or two celery stalks
- Take one half of an English cucumber
- Juice one lemon
- One half cup of your best unsweetened almond milk (You can also replace the milk with water if you cannot find unsweetened almond milk

Blend completely and then stop the blender to add in three to four ice cubes and then blend for 30 seconds.

F) Peanut Butter Oatmeal

Directions: Not only is this delicious, it is a favorite of athletes for the energy it provides. Microwave ½ cup of steel cut oats combined with ¾ of a cup, of unsweetened almond milk for three minutes. Place 2 teaspoons of organic peanut butter on top and stir evenly. Once it is thoroughly mixed, sprinkle on ¼ teaspoon of an unsweetened cocoa powder to give it that extra zip. Mix it well and enjoy.

G) Quinoa Breakfast Cup

Directions: If you haven't tried quinoa, now is the time. This ancient grain was a staple of the South American tribes who needed plenty of energy to complete their runs from village to village.

Start by cooking one cup of quinoa and put it in the fridge overnight. In the morning, take a mixing bowl and add 2 cups of your favorite brand of plain Greek yogurt. You will need ¾ of one lime skin, shredded. Mix this well and then clean and cut 10 strawberries and 2 peeled kiwi fruit, although some people prefer to leave the skin on for extra fiber.

You can put this together in a clear glass or jar if you want the kids getting excited to eat it, or in a small bowl. Start by putting in a layer of quinoa in the bottom, followed by a layer of the yogurt mix and a layer of fruit and continue to do layers until finished. This actually looks really delicious when you do it in a clear glass container.

Are you enjoying this book?
If so, I'd be really happy if you could leave a short review on Amazon, it means a lot to me!

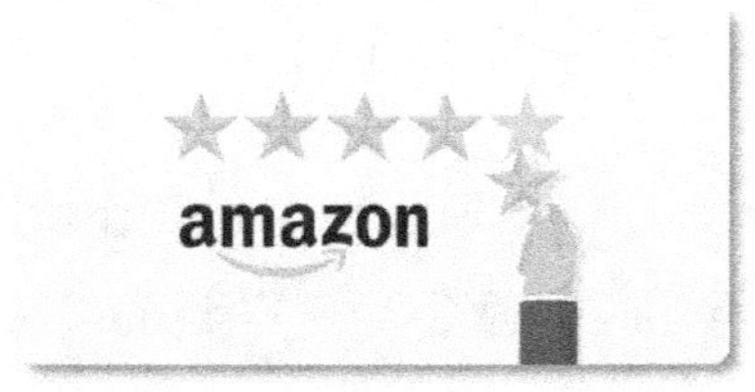

Thank you.

A)   Baked Sardines and Vegetables

Directions: Try to find fresh sardines or plain canned sardines for this dish. You will need:
- 10 to 12 sardines
- 1 eggplant
- 1 large red pepper
- 1 purple or Spanish onion
- ½ cup of cherry tomatoes
- 2 zucchini
- 1 tablespoon virgin olive oil
- 2 diced cloves of garlic
- 1 teaspoon of red wine vinegar
- Black pepper and sea salt to taste

To start, use a large mixing bowl for your chopped/sliced eggplant, red pepper, zucchini, cherry tomatoes, onion and garlic. Mix it completely and then add the oil, vinegar sea salt and pepper. Again mix it thoroughly. While preheating your oven to 400 degrees, take a large baking tray and line it with parchment paper to avoid sticking. Add your mixture and when the oven is ready, bake for 20 minutes.

In another small tray, place the sardines and brush them with virgin olive oil, then season with salt and pepper. Once your vegetable mixture has cooked for 20 minutes, remove from the oven and layer the coated sardines on top. Place back in the oven for an additional 20 minutes and enjoy.

B)   Kale and Spinach Salad With Cherry Tomatoes

Directions: Many people find kale to be somewhat bitter, so combining it with spinach and seasonings, is the way to go.
- ½ of a kale bind. Fresh kale comes wrapped with a small cord, so use only ½
- ½ of a bundle of spinach
- 1 carrot
- 1 cucumber
- 1 yellow bell pepper
- minced garlic

To start off, clean your kale and spinach carefully and then take the kale and run a rolling pin over it before finely chopping. This helps to break down the kale as it is a thick leaf vegetable. Dice up your carrots, cucumber, bell pepper and add this to a bowl. Many recipes call for powered garlic but fresh is much better for you. You can purchase small grinders that are perfect for garlic and many people grind up huge bundles of garlic, put them in a jar and refrigerate. Once you have the garlic processed, add in 1 teaspoon to your mixing bowl and stir completely.

Dressings for this salad are optional. Many people just drizzle virgin olive oil over it. If you want to dazzle your taste buds, you can make a homemade dressing:
- ½ cup of balsamic vinegar
- ½ cup of pure virgin olive oil
- ½ teaspoon of oregano
- Squeeze the juice from one lemon
- ¼ teaspoon each of sea salt, black pepper and lemon pepper

You will want to put this in your fridge overnight to cool, so the night before, take the mixture and put it into a mason jar or something similar that can be sealed tight. Shake it well and place in the fridge. Before using on your salad, be sure to give it another good shake to make sure it is thoroughly mixed and then add to your salad in moderation.

C)   Quinoa and Salmon Lunch Treat

Directions: For this super healthy lunch you will need:
- 2 cups Quinoa
- 2-3 Salmon fillets
- 1 White onion
- 1 diced Tomato

- 1 cup of Spinach
- Salt and pepper to taste
- 2 tablespoons of Balsamic vinegar
- 1 tablespoon of Virgin olive oil
- 2 tablespoons of Dijon mustard

Let's start by making our sugar free dressing. In a small mix bowl, add 3 tablespoons of virgin olive oil, 2 tablespoons of balsamic vinegar, 1 to 2 tablespoons of Dijon mustard, and a full teaspoon of minced garlic. Get your whisk and blend this all nicely.

In a frying pan, heat the virgin olive oil and pan sear the salmon filets for 5 minutes. While this is taking place, use another mixing bowl to put in your 2 cups of previously cooked and cooled quinoa. Add in one diced tomato, approximately 4 cups of chopped spinach, your onion and salt/pepper. Everyone's taste buds are different, so if like balsamic vinegar, you can add a splash and then stir your mixture.
Once your salmon is cooked and has cooled sufficiently, use a fork to break it up and then stir it into the salad mixture. Top with your homemade salad dressing.

D)   Tuna and Spinach Salad

Directions: You cannot go wrong with tuna, it is so simple to use in many different recipes. For this easy salad, you need:

- 1 can of white tuna
- 1 cup of spinach
- ½ cup of cherry tomatoes, sliced in halves
- ¼ teaspoon of sea salt and ¼ teaspoon of black pepper.
- 1 tablespoon of fresh lemon juice
- 1/3 cup of plain Greek yogurt

Combine all the ingredients in a mixing bowl and enjoy.

E)   3 Bean Salad

Directions: First of, let's talk about putting the work in. It is recommended that you buy your dry beans, soak them overnight in water and then cook them the next day. Whew! Okay, if you use canned beans, put them in a strainer and flush them thoroughly with water. What do we use?
- 1 cup of chick peas
- 1 cup of kidney beans
- 1 cup of pinto beans
- 2 celery stalks chopped
- 4 diced green onion stalks and bulbs
- ¼ cup of virgin olive oil
- 2 tablespoons of balsamic vinegar

- 1 tablespoon of Dijon mustard
- Your choice of ¼ teaspoon of paprika, or chilli powder.

You will need one large mixing bowl for your beans, celery, and green onion. Combine the olive oil, balsamic vinegar, mustard and paprika or chilli powder. Stir it well. Once you have thoroughly mixed the ingredients in the large bowl, add the homemade dressing. This salad is best if cooled in the fridge first. You can sprinkle parsley on top of your bowl of bean salad, if desired.

F)   Sliced Steak Salad

Directions: Having some protein with your veggies is one way of staying full and not craving sugar. Here is a simple recipe for beef lovers.

- 1 small piece of a good cut of beef
- 2 cups of spinach
- ¾ cup of halved cherry tomatoes
- ¼ cup of purple onion
- ½ cup of pure virgin olive oil
- ¼ cup of fresh lemon juice
- ¼ teaspoon of sea salt and same for the black pepper

Slice your piece of steak into thin strips and stir fry in olive oil until just a bit of pink can be seen.

Combine your spinach which is finely chopped, the tomatoes and finely diced onion in a big mixing bowl. In a small mixing cup or bowl, combine the olive oil, lemon juice and salt/pepper. Stir it completely. Once your steak strips have cooled, add them to the salad bowl and top with your home made dressing.

G)   Bacon and Avocado Salad

Directions: Yes bacon is normally eaten at breakfast but hey bacon is yummy. You will want to check the packages to make sure it is sugar free or even substitute sugar free turkey bacon.

- 4 to 6 cooked strips of bacon
- 2 cored avocado diced up
- 6 boiled eggs, normally hardboiled but you can go with just a soft center
- 2 tablespoons of plain Greek yogurt
- 2 teaspoons of fresh lemon juice
- ½ cup of freshly chopped cilantro-substitute green onion if you do not like cilantro
- Sprinkled sea salt and pepper on the finished salad

In a salad bowl, start by putting in your avocado nicely chopped up, followed by the eggs sliced up. Mix in the bacon after cutting it into small pieces.

Add the yogurt, lemon juice and cilantro and gently mix the bowl. After putting your desired helping into a dish, lightly season with salt and pepper.

7 Main Dishes Recipes

A)   3 Bean Vegetarian Chilli

Directions: With this type of dinner, many people alter the spice according to the season. That means less spice in summer and then kick it up in the winter. We will go over the spice as a basic heat, nothing flame throwing. For the beans, again it is recommended to use dried beans, soaked overnight and then cooked.

- 2 cups of chickpeas
- 2 cups of kidney beans
- 2 cups of garbanzo beans
- 1 cup of frozen corn
- 1 diced Spanish onion
- 4 cups of diced or blended fresh tomatoes
- 2 teaspoons of chilli powder
- 2 teaspoons of cumin
- 2 chopped bell peppers of any color
- Pinch of salt and ½ teaspoon of black pepper

- 1 cup of homemade beef stock preferred
- 1 teaspoon of minced garlic

In a large sized pot, add in some virgin olive oil and stir in the onion and garlic. Once that is cooked, mix in all your beans and corn, stir well and put in the tomatoes and stock.

Add your chilli powder, cumin, salt and pepper. Cook on medium heat for an hour and then reduce to low for ½ to 1 hour.

Note: Depending on where you live, winter can be extremely cold. Kick this up to toasty hot by chopping 2 Thai chilli peppers and stir fry that with the onion and garlic. This will release the chilli juice and give you a really nice and spicy vegetable chilli.

B)	Baked Chicken With Trees

Directions: Okay we aren't really cooking trees but when you cut up the broccoli and cauliflower into small florets, well they look like miniature trees.
- 1 head each of cauliflower and broccoli
- 2 to 4 chicken breasts sliced down the center.
- ¼ cup of virgin olive oil
- 3 teaspoons of minced garlic
- 3 teaspoons of turmeric

Start by cutting the cauliflower and broccoli into bite sized florets. Place them in a large mixing bowl and add the olive oil, turmeric and minced garlic. You can sprinkle the desired amount of sea salt and black pepper here, if you wish to add it in.

In a separate bowl, place your chicken and drizzle it with olive oil, a dash of turmeric.

Set the oven to 450 degrees and use a paper towel to grease it with some olive oil. Place your cauliflower/broccoli mixture on the tray and spread them around evenly. Cook for 20 minutes and use a spatula to flip them at the 10 minute mark for even cooking.

Reduce your heat to 400 and move the florets around to make room for the chicken. Cook for approximately 15 minutes and remove. When serving this, you can go paleo and add chopped walnuts as a topping.

C)   Slow Cooker Diced Chicken and Beans

Directions: You have to love all the slow cooker recipes out there. Set it and forget it.

- 2 skinless chicken breasts
- 3 large tomatoes

- 1 Spanish onion
- 2 cups of chick peas
- 2 cups of pinto beans
- 3 teaspoons of cumin
- 2 cups of homemade chicken broth
- 3 teaspoons of minced garlic
- 1 teaspoon of oregano
- ½ teaspoon each of sea salt and black pepper

As normal, soak and cook your beans first. The chicken is diced up and it does not need to be browned. Put all the ingredients into your slow cooker and set on low for 8 hours.

D)   Slow Cooked Pork Tenderloin

Directions: This is a way to make juicy pork as many people find pork to be a bit dry.

- 2 lbs of pork tenderloin
- 1 diced onion
- 1 tablespoon of minced garlic
- 2 teaspoons of Italian seasoning
- 2 tablespoons of virgin olive oil
- ½ cup of balsamic vinegar
- ½ cup of water or vegetable broth
- 1 teaspoon each of sea salt and black pepper

The way to get going on this is making a dry seasoning rub with the Italian seasoning, pepper and salt. Mix it together in a bowl.
Put the pork tenderloin on a large plate and thoroughly rub the seasoning over it.

Unlike chicken breast, pork needs a little help before it goes into the crock pot. Start by putting the balsamic vinegar and garlic in your frying pan. Cook it on medium heat while stirring constantly. Once your garlic is cooked, add in the pork tenderloin. You want to pan sear the pork while basting it in the vinegar/garlic mixture.

Transfer your pork to the slow cooker and add the juice you created in the fry pan. Next add in the water/vegetable broth. Note: The vegetable broth is much tastier but you need to make homemade.

Cook your pork for 3 hours on high or 7-8 hours on low. Pork needs to be fully cooked, so use a fork and knife to cut into it and check or if you have a meat thermometer, look for it to be cooked when it reaches 170 degrees.

This is similar to pulled pork, so slicing it up after it finished will be a snap.

E)   Slow Cooker Beef and Horseradish

Directions: If you have never had horseradish before, it is like a spice. Many people note that when they eat it, they get a warming sensation in the nostrils. Beef and horseradish is yummy.

- 2 pounds of stewing beef already cubed
- 1 teaspoon of paprika
- 1 teaspoon of minced ginger
- 1 teaspoon of virgin olive oil
- 3 finely diced purple onions
- 1 tablespoon of minced garlic
- 2 teaspoons of Dijon mustard
- 1 cup of diced button mushrooms
- 2 teaspoons of corn flower
- 2 cups of homemade beef stock
- 1 even tablespoon of minced horseradish

We want to pan sear our beef, so we start by putting the paprika, flour and ginger in a bowl. Add in the beef and stir thoroughly.
In the fry pan, add your virgin olive oil and pan sear the beef mixture.

Transfer the beef to the slow cooker and add in the minced horseradish, mustard, onions and stock. Cook on low for 6 hours before adding in your mushrooms and continue to cook for 2 more hours.

There you have a nice tasty stew with a very different flavor.

F)   Slow Cooked Balsamic Chicken Thighs

Directions: This is a great dish for those who want protein but find white chicken meat too dry, no matter how it is cooked.

- 8 boneless thighs with the skin removed
- ½ cup of balsamic vinegar
- 1 teaspoon of minced garlic
- 1 teaspoon of dried basil
- 1 tablespoon of virgin olive oil
- 1 small diced onion
- ½ teaspoon each of sea salt and black pepper

In a big mixing bowl lay out the thighs. Sprinkle the garlic, basil, onion, salt and pepper over the chicken. Take a few moments to roll the chicken around in the spice mixture getting an even coat.

Take the crock pot and add the oil and the first half of the balsamic vinegar. Put the chicken on top and drizzle the rest of the vinegar over it.

Set it to high and cook for three hours.

G)   Steamed Halibut With Vegetables

Directions: This is super easy to make and steaming your vegetables is much better than cooking them in water.

- 4 fillets of halibut
- 1 full head of broccoli, cut into bite sized florets
- 3 zucchini sliced thin
- 4 teaspoons of virgin olive oil
- 2-3 tablespoons of chopped parsley
- Pinch of sea salt and pepper
- 2 lemons

You will need a big sauce pan and a steamer that fits snugly. Put enough water in the sauce pan, so that it is just below the steamer. Bring it to a boil and add in the vegetables. As they steam, check them for texture. Some people prefer their vegetables steamed but still with a bit of crunch.

Once you are happy with the vegetables, put them into a large mixing bowl and sprinkle a pinch of salt over them.

Check the water level in the saucepan and while it gets up to boil again, rub the fish with a pinch of salt and pepper.

Add your fish to the steamer and check it after about five minutes. If it is not does come apart easy with a fork, then cook for another 2 to 3 minutes.

After your fish is done, transfer it to the dinner plates with the vegetables and drizzle the virgin olive oil over it. Your parsley should be finely chopped and now you can sprinkle it over the food. The lemons are optional. If desired, squeeze one half lemon over the fish and vegetables.

7 Recipes to Replace Traditional Desserts

A)   Peanut Butter-Banana-Oatmeal Cookies
Directions:

-1/3 of a cup organic peanut butter
-2 bananas use ripe, not green
-1 teaspoon vanilla
-2 tablespoons soy milk
-2 tablespoons maple syrup
-2 and 1/2 cups quick-cooking plain oatmeal
-A pinch of cinnamon
-1/4 cup flour

Grab a large mixing bowl and put the bananas in first. Use a fork or whatever works best to turn them into mashed bananas. Add in the peanut butter, maple syrup and vanilla...mixing it up nicely. Finish off by putting in the rest of the ingredients and mix it all together evenly.

Use a tablespoon to scoop up the mixture and place each ball on an ungreased cookie tray.

Use the back of the spoon to flatten slightly. Bake at 350 degrees for 15 minutes.

B)   Shortbread Cookies

Description: Shortbread cookies are plain and simple, yet they taste great.

- ¼ cup of Erythritol
- 1 and 1/3 cup of almond flour
- 1 cup of unsalted butter, not melted but at room temperature
- ½ teaspoon of vanilla essence
- 1/8 of teaspoon sea salt

Mix all the ingredient together with a hand blender, and then hand roll into small balls. Put them on a plate and into the fridge for 15 minutes.

You will need a good sized cookie tray covered with parchment paper. After the cookie dough has been in the fridge for 10 minute, preheat the oven at 350 degrees.

Lay out your cookie balls on the tray and gentle depress them with a fork. Cook for 10 minutes and check. The tops should be golden brown and if required, leave in the oven for another minute.

C)   Lemon Cake

Description: This is a beautiful cake with a lovely lemon flavor from real lemons.

- You need a 16 ounce box of sugar free yellow cake mix
- 3 eggs
- ¾ cup of water
- 1/3 cup of vegetable oil
- 3 lemons
- ¼ cup of sugar free strawberry preserves
- 2 cups of fresh strawberries

In a large mixing bowl, put in the yellow cake mix, water, eggs, and vegetable oil. Take your lemons and using a scraper, zest the peels and add those. Cut and squeeze the zested lemons into a bowl, removing the seeds. Add this to the big mixing bowl and using a hand mixer, stir it up for 3 minutes or until thoroughly mixed.

Using a large steel muffin tray, spoon the mixture into the greased individual cups, leaving room at the top.

Bake for 20 minutes at 350 degrees. While this is baking, you will make a strawberry topping.

In a saucepan, add ¼ cup of sugar free strawberry preserves and heat/stir for on medium. You are looking for it to turn slightly liquid, before adding in the fresh strawberries and stir the whole mixture for another five minutes. Set it to low and when the cake mix is done, remove from the oven. Let them cool before removing and putting into individual small bowls. Before serving, spoon the strawberry mixture over the cake.

D)   Sugar Free Banana Cream Pie

Directions: Banana cream pie is very popular due to the texture and taste. Using a graham cracker crust enhances this pie.

- 1 and ½ cups of sugar free graham crackers
- 6 tablespoons of unsalted butter
- 1/3 of cup of erythritol as your sweetener

- 1 ounce bar of cream cheese-let it soften up first
- 1 sugar free whipped topping
- 1 box of sugar free banana pudding. Look for a 4 servings size

We will start with the pie crust and then let it cool while we make the filling.

For the graham crackers, they need to be crushed and you can use your food processor for this. If you don't have one, you need thick zip lock bags and a rolling pin, to crush the crackers evenly.

Get your pie plate ready and if you don't have a non-stick, you will need to grease it to avoid sticking. Find a large mixing bowl and start by putting in your crushed graham crackers.

Put in your erythritol next and give it all a good stir, while melting the butter in a small sauce pan. Once the butter is ready add it to the mixture and stir.

Now it is time to test the mixture for how it sticks together. We need it sticky enough that when applied to the pie plate and patted down, it won't fall apart. Get a handful of the mixture and make a ball. If it appears this is going to crumble, then start adding tiny amounts of water, or melted butter to the mixture until you get the right consistency.

Once you have it just right, put it into the pie plate and form the crust. Your oven should be preheated to 375 degrees. Approximately 10 minutes in the oven should give you a nice pie crust.

In your mixer or large bowl, you put in the cream cheese and start blending it, followed by half the whipped topping. The last item to go in is your lemon mix and then continue to blend.

Spread this mixture evenly into your pie crust and smooth it out. Next step is to put it in the fridge for 3 hours. When you take it, use the rest of the whipped topping to spread over the pie.

E)	Peanut Butter and Jam Bars

Description: Yes it is true, kids love peanut butter and jelly sandwiches. Well the kid in you is going to love these bars.

- 1 and ½ cups of all-purpose flower
- ¾ cup of erythritol as your sugar alternative
- 1 cup of sugar free peanut butter
- ½ teaspoon of baking powder
- ¾ cup of sugar free jam

- 1 egg
- 1 teaspoon of vanilla extract
- ½ cup of unsalted butter or vegan butter if you prefer
- ¾ cup of chopped salted peanuts

All right let's get to it. Get out your large cookie tray and line it with parchment paper. It is also advised that you give the paper a quick spray with your best non-stick spray, as these cookies are sticky starting out.

In your large mixing bowl put in the erythritol and butter. If hand blending, make sure you mix it thoroughly.

In a separate bowl, whisk your flour and baking powder completely.

Your mixed bowl should be completely whisked and now you can add in that one egg, peanut butter and vanilla.
Your mixed flour and baking powder is going into the mixing bowl next, but be sure to add a bit at a time, mix, then add some more to get it completely mixed together.

Now comes the fun part because we are going to construct the bars by putting one half of our mixture in the fridge to cool, while prepping the other half with the other ingredients.

Take the remainder of mix that is in your bowl and spread it evenly over the greased parchment paper.

Your jam comes next and you need to spread it over the pan mixture and coat it evenly.

Once the mixture in your fridge is completely cool, remove it and start building your bars.

The trick here is to get small amounts of the cold mixture and hand flatten them before placing them on top of the jam. Trying to spread it will just move the jam all around. Once you have your cold mixture on top, sprinkle the chopped peanuts on top and place the tray in the oven. Bake for 50 minutes at 325 degrees.

You need to let the bars cool off before cutting them into squares.

F)   A Tasty Sugar Free Blueberry Ice Cream

Directions: Blueberries are delicious and everyone loves ice cream. There is no need to give it up on the Sugar Detox, because sugar free ice cream is a snap to make.

- 1 and ¼ cup of coconut cream
- 1 teaspoon of vanilla extract
- 2 and ½ cups of frozen blueberries
- 1 and ½ tablespoons of erythritol

For this recipe, you need either a food processor or a heavy duty blender.

As mentioned, this is super simple. Just put all your ingredients into the processor/blender and mix until you get the thickness that you like. Since the blueberries are frozen, this should be cold and thick enough to eat right away.

G)   Delightful Sugar Free Brownies

These brownies will help those who crave chocolate and brownies are always a hit with the family.

- 1 teaspoon of baking powder
- 1 cup of all-purpose flour
- ¾ cup of unsweetened cocoa powder
- 1 and ½ cups of erythritol sugar replacement
- 1 cup of unsalted butter
- 3 eggs
- 2 teaspoons of vanilla extract
- 1 cup of sugar free chocolate chips

You'll need a square baking pan, lined with parchment paper. You may find it easier to let the parchment paper fold over the edges, for easier removal of the brownies.

In a large mixing bowl, blend the erythritol and butter. In a smaller bowl, whisk together your flour, baking powder and the unsweetened cocoa.

Now we combine the dry mixture to a large mixing bowl and whisk it all together. Add the eggs, one at a time and whisk those to mix it completely.

You will put in the vanilla next, mix it well and then do the same with the sugar free chocolate chips.

The oven gets preheated to 325 degrees, while transferring your mixture to the square pan. Use a spatula to smooth it out in the pan. Bake for 25 minutes. As with any cake or brownie mixture, timing is everything. Check your brownies by inserting a toothpick and see if anything clings. This means it may need a bit more time to cook.

Remove and let it cool before cutting into squares.

7 Snacks To Keep Sugar Craving Away

We all get hungry between meals. Here are 7 simple snacks to keep you off the sugar.

Carrots and Hummus

Some people use baby carrots but there is some controversy as to what these carrots may be soaked in. For health's sake, it is better to go with organic small carrots. These are easier to consume than hard large carrots. To make this a tasty snack, you need to purchase hummus. Hummus is primarily made from chickpeas that are ground up. Do a bit of research and look for brands that are five stars, so you know you are getting good quality.

Popcorn Anyone?

People who love popcorn can get a good quality one by using Newman's Own Butter Microwave Popcorn. Newman's is a little more expensive but great quality. Eat in moderation.

Spicy Chickpeas

Try this spicy snack you can make at home Spicy chickpeas can be baked and are nice and crunchy. Soak a bag of dried chickpeas overnight in a bowl. Drain and mix in a bowl with a dash of virgin olive oil. Add in 1 teaspoon of cumin, 1 and ½ teaspoons of cayenne pepper and salt and pepper to taste. Remember everyone's spice level is different, so feel free to adjust the cumin and cayenne accordingly. Spread on a cookie sheet and bake at 400 degrees for 35 to 40 minutes. You want these to be crunchy, so turn off the oven and leave the tray inside. As the heat dies down, the peas will let out the remaining moisture and become crunchy. Once your oven has cooled off completely, remove and enjoy.

Baked Tortilla Chips With Homemade Salsa

Homemade salsa is the best. To be honest, store bought salsa is not hot to some folks, even when the jar reads," Hot!"

For the chips, we buy a 12 ounce bag of corn chips. If the chips are large, you can break them into smaller pieces, to make them go around. In a bowl, put 1 tablespoon of pure virgin olive oil and 3 tablespoons of freshly squeezed lime juice. Whisk until blended. To coat the chips, you can spray this mixture on or use a brush.

In a 2nd bowl, mix 1 teaspoon of cumin, 1 teaspoon of chilli powder and 1 teaspoon of salt. Sprinkle ½ of this on the chips and bake for 8 minutes at 350 degrees. Flip the chips and sprinkle the remainder of the spice mixture, baking for another 8 minute. The chips should be crispy.

To make the homemade salsa for dipping, put the following into a blender and mix thoroughly.

- 8 large tomatoes, chopped
- 1 cup of diced white onion
- 2 cloves of garlic minced
- ½ cup of freshly chopped cilantro
- Juice of one freshly squeezed lime
- ½ teaspoon of sea salt
- ½ teaspoon of cumin
- 1 teaspoon of virgin olive oil
- 1 diced red pepper
- 1 to 2 finely diced jalapeno seeds removed or if you want hotter, use 1-2 Thai red chilli with seeds removed.

Blend it all together and put in the fridge to cool before dipping your chips.

Sesame Date Rolls You Can Eat On The Go!

When you are heading to the office or the gym, try one or two of these sesame date rolls, to keep you on the move. Here is what you need:

- 8 ounces of dried dates
- ¼ of toasted sesame seeds
- ¼ cup of chopped walnuts
- ½ cup of whole raw almonds
- 1 cup of hot water
- ½ cup of unsweetened shredded coconut
- 1 tablespoon of coconut oil
- ¾ of a teaspoon ground cardamom
- ¼ of a teaspoon of cinnamon powder
- 1 teaspoon of vanilla extract
- ¼ of a teaspoon of sea salt

Start this recipe by placing the dates in a small mixing bowl, adding the hot water to soften them. Be sure the water covers the dates and leave it for 15 minutes.

In your food processor, toss in the dates after you have drained the juice off into a bowl. Add 2 tablespoons from your toasted sesame seeds and everything else. Set the processor to pulse and go through a few cycles. Check to see if anything is sticking to the sides, if so unplug the processor and use a spatula to scrape the sides. Look at the thickness of your mixture. If it appears to be too thick, you can a few drips of the drained date juice from that bowl you set aside on the counter.

The final step is log rolling. Not those big logs in the river. ☺ We are talking about putting all your dough onto a large piece of parchment paper. Grease up your hands and proceed to form the dough mixture into a long roll. Think of the cardboard piece inside your paper towel, when you are stumped about size. Once that is done, start taking the rest of the sesame seeds and sprinkling/gently pressing them into the outside of the log. When this step is complete, roll the log up using the parchment paper and twist the ends. This log goes into your fridge for two hours. Remove and slice pieces in your desired thickness.

Avocado Pudding

It seems avocado goes with everything, including dates. Who knew? Try this yummy recipe for a snack.

- 20 dried dates without pits
- 1 large avocado, ripe is better
- 1 ripe banana
- ½ cup of almond butter
- ½ cup of unsweetened cocoa powder

- ¼ cup of almond milk
- ¼ of a teaspoon of sea salt.

We start this off by soaking the dates in a pot of hot water, fully covering the dates. After the dates have soaked for 15 minutes turn on high and bring to a boil while giving it a stir. Once the dates being to boil, lower the stove to low and let simmer for 20 minutes.
From here we transfer the dates and juice to a food processor and blend until nice and smooth.

Add in all your other ingredient and continue to blend. Stop and check to see if anything is sticking to the sides and if so, use a spatula to scrape it down. Always unplug the processor before doing this.

Once everything is nicely blended, move it into individual containers. Small glass containers with the plastic lids work well. Put in the fridge for 1 to 2 hours.

Turmeric Cashews With Tasty Coconut Shreds

Why have just plain cashews to snack on, when you can get the health benefit of the powerful spice known as turmeric.

Easy as pie to make.

-1 and ½ teaspoons of coconut oil
- 1 teaspoon of turmeric
- Just a thumb and forefinger pinch of sea salt and black pepper
- ½ cup of coconut flakes
- 2 cups of cashews

Use a cookie tray lined with parchment paper. Put everything except the coconut flakes on the tray and hand mix. Preheat the oven to 350 degrees. Once the oven is ready, place the cookie tray in for 10 minutes. Flip the mixture around with a steel spatula after the 5 minute mark and when 8 minutes is up, sprinkle in the coconut flakes. Check the mixture during this time so it doesn't burn, you just want it golden on top.

Let cool and snack away.

Conclusion... or not?

After completing this eBook, you should have a new lifestyle. One that sees you happy and fit, without gobbling down pounds of refined sugar products.

Many people wonder what happens if they go back to the way they were. It can happen and you need to make some adjustments.
In most cases, a relapse happens due to a very stressful event such as job loss, divorce or the death of a loved one.

In this time, you need to do self-talk and explain that relapsing will not help at all and make life worse. You direct yourself to up the amount of serotonin and dopamine activities each and every day. Relapsing is not the end of the world, it is your brain telling you something is a bit off and you need to fix it. So don't kick yourself in the butt.

You may find that due to stress or the lack of proper exercise, you need some support. Don't be afraid to get recommendations from your doctor or find a workout buddy/trainer. Analyze the issue and make a new action plan to conquer this.

UNEXPECTED BONUS!

Boost Your Immune System – Trainig Guide
FREE FOR YOU!

Continue reading next page...

Boost Your Immune System Training Guide

Introduction

Your immune system is vital for preventing and fighting off diseases. This is especially important with the current coronavirus pandemic. Our lifestyles usually dictate the health of our immune system and if you want to improve this vital component of your body then you need to be prepared to make some difficult changes.

Boosting your immune system starts by understanding what it does and how it works. We have a chapter on this that explains everything in a simple to understand way. Once you know how much your immune system protects you, it will be easier for you to make the changes that you need to make.

Some things in life cause harm to your immune system and if you indulge in these then you need to stop. Smoking and drinking alcohol are high on the list here which will probably not surprise you. But there are other things that you need to avoid as well that we cover in detail.

The right diet will provide the nutrients and vitamins that your immune system needs to stay in tip top condition and work hard for you. Changing your diet is a big step to take, but if you are eating the wrong things then you need to do this for the sake of your immune system.

There are supplements available that can provide essential vitamins and minerals that perhaps your diet cannot. We provide you with all of the information that you need to know about supplements in this guide.

Stress can negatively impact your immune system and we have a whole chapter dedicated to how you can reduce the stress in your life. Exercising regularly and getting the right amount of sleep are also very important and we cover this off for you as well.

Keeping your body clear of toxins is something else that will help your immune system and we have some great detoxification techniques for you in this guide. Finally we explain why essential oils are beneficial for your immune system and the best ones to use.

Why you need to boost your immune system

Do you always find that when the colds and flu do the rounds you seem to get them while others around you are unaffected? If this is the case for you then you should definitely take steps to strengthen your immune system.

Most people seem to pay more attention to their immune systems during the winter months, when colds and the flu are at peak levels. But you need to understand that your immune system works hard for you every day of the year and it does a lot more than just protect you from colds and flu.

Your Immune System is very Precious

Every one of us has this wonderful thing called an immune system designed to keep us healthy and well. It protects us 24/7 without us even realizing it. There are a number of things that you can do to boost your immune system as you will discover in later chapters of this guide.

But there are also a number of things that can damage your immune system and its ability to protect you against bacteria, pathogens and viruses. At the time of writing this guide, the world is gripped by the coronavirus pandemic so having a strong immune system is vital.

Do you have a Weak Immune System?

A lot of people have weak immune systems and don't even know it. If you do have a weakened immune system then you must do something about it fast. There are a few signs that you can watch out for to see if your immune system is weak:

Diseases that Weaken the Immune System

There are some diseases that will weaken your immune system. Some of these are really well known such as AIDS and HIV. These are auto-immune diseases that can significantly damage your immune system unless you get the right treatment.

Some cancers will weaken your immune system too. There are also people that are born with disorders affecting their immune systems that make them more deficient than other people's. At the time of writing there was no cure for this type of disorder so anyone that has this must manage it for life.

Getting the same Infections over and over

If you get the same infections over and over again on a regular basis then this is definitely a sign of a weakened immune system. For people with normal or strong immune systems, getting these infections will only occur a small number of times in their life.

To be more specific, do you regularly suffer from a strep throat or pneumonia? If so then this probably means that your immune system is weaker than it should be. Another sign is frequent problems with your digestive system.

It is also possible that more common ailments such as diarrhea, a lack of appetite and stomach pains on a regular basis could point to a weakened immune system. A large proportion of your immune system covers your digestive system, so if all is not well here then your immune system could be weak.

Low Energy Levels

In some people, low energy levels are an indicator that there is a weakness in their immune system. The reason for this is that your body is spending much more energy than it should do ensuring that your immune system works as hard as possible for you. If you are sleeping well then a weak immune system could be the reason that your energy levels are down.

If you are Sick right now can you still Boost your Immune System?

Yes you certainly can and you must. Your immune system is still working hard for you while you are sick, not only tackling the sickness that you have but also ensuring that no new diseases arise. So it needs all the help that you can give it.

If you follow all of the practices recommended in this guide (which we strongly recommend) and you do get sick, this does not mean that the practices are flawed. It just means that something slipped through the net so you need to carry on the good work if you are sick.

If you are concerned whether your immune system is in good shape and do not want to test it by being exposed to a disease (not a good idea), then we strongly recommend that you have a blood test specifically for your immune system.

The immune system blood test will check the amount of white blood cells that you have. This is very important as these white blood cells fight diseases and take out certain cells to protect you. If your white blood cell count is low then your immune system will be weak.

Another thing that a blood test will do is check for antibodies or immunoglobulin. These are vital for your immune system because they are proteins designed specifically to attack different diseases.

If you are a pregnant woman then you can have a blood test to check if their unborn child has an autoimmune disease. Treatment can be administered if this is the case, otherwise a child can be in real danger. Autoimmune diseases can be passed through blood so there are often genetics involved.

In order to boost your immune system in the best way you need to know where you are starting from. Do you have a normal immune system for your age (in later years your immune system deteriorates) or do you have a weak immune system right now?

In the next chapter we will discuss how your immune system works...

How Your Immune System Works

Don't worry, you do not have to be a doctor to understand this chapter. We have kept it as simple as possible so that anyone can gain a good understanding of what their immune system really does and how it works.

What does your Immune System do?

The purpose of your immune system is to protect you from foreign invasions that can harm you. These foreign invaders are called "antigens". An antigen could be a parasite, bacteria, fungi or viruses (such as the coronavirus).

Whenever these antigens are discovered in your body they will trigger your immune system. Once kicked into action, your immune system will do everything possible to destroy these antigens using a variety of methods. It really is an amazing system that you need to take care of all of your life.

Your Innate Immune System

The human immune system is divided into two categories:

1. Innate
2. Adaptive

Think of your innate immune system as the "first responder" to any antigens that find their way into your body. Your innate immune system is made up of your skin, the cells within your immune system and certain chemicals in your blood.

Your skin really is your first line of defense because it provides a barrier on the surface of your body to prevent bacteria and viruses getting inside. If you are wondering why there is so much emphasis on washing your hands with the coronavirus pandemic, it is a way to destroy antigens before they can enter your body.

The Cells of your Immune System

Your immune system contains vital immune cells. Some of these cells are more selective than the others when it comes to defending against certain antigens. There are 3 main types of immune system cells:

1. T Cells
2. B Cells
3. Phagocytes

The purpose of T cells is to regulate your immune cells. It can activate the cells or eliminate them. If there are abnormal cells in your body or some that are infected with antigens then T cells will kill them. They are "killer cells".

The B cells in your immune system will activate the necessary antibodies. These antibodies are proteins that have the sole purpose of destroying antigens in your bloodstream. B cells perform a vital role.

Phagocytes are larger white cells that basically eat antigens. You will find phagocytes in tissue and blood. If you notice some inflammation in your body this is very likely to be phagocytes at work. When your immune system needs to send phagocytes to a part of your body it can cause inflammation to increase the flow of blood.

Your Adaptive Immune System

Your adaptive immune system has a very important role as it remembers any past antigen attacks you have encountered. It uses this information to attack these same antigens in a more effective way.

You will have had at least one vaccine as a child. The reason that vaccines work is that they trigger your adaptive immune system, so that whenever one of the antigens in the vaccine is encountered again it will know how to deal with it in the most effective way.

Your adaptive immune system will remember specific antigens and then dispatch the appropriate immune cells to destroy them. This is a fast and effective process which prevents a buildup of the antigens in your body.

Your Lymphatic System

You have another critical system in your body which helps prevent you from becoming sick and this is your lymphatic system. It comprises nodes, vessels and tissues that assist your body to eliminate toxins and any other substances that can cause you harm.

Your lymphatic system circulates lymph fluid through your body. This contains white blood cells (similar to the B cells and T cells we discussed above).

That wasn't too painful was it?

So there you have it – a lay guide to your complex immune system. We believe that it is very important that you understand what your immune system is and how it works. This will help you when it comes to avoiding the things that can harm your immune system and doing the things that will help to boost it.

In the next chapter we will discuss the things that you need to avoid to protect your immune system...

Avoid These Things to Protect Your Immune System

The secret to boosting your immune system is to lead as healthy a lifestyle as you can. A lot of people will adopt a healthy lifestyle when they are sick, but we strongly recommend that you adopt a healthy lifestyle all of the time so that you can avoid getting sick in the first place.

Nobody said that this was going to be easy. If you have a pretty unhealthy lifestyle at the moment then it is going to take a lot of effort and persistence on your part to make the transition to a healthy lifestyle.

You now know how vital your immune system is for your health and wellbeing. So keep this uppermost in your mind when you are cutting out the bad things and bringing in the good things. A healthy lifestyle is best for not only your physical health, but your mental health as well.

In the first chapter we looked at things that can weaken your immune system such as auto-immune diseases. These can be treated and help you to build up your immune system. There are other things that you can certainly avoid to prevent damage to your immune system as well, so let's take a look at these.

Smoking

You just knew that this was going to come up didn't you? There are many health risks with smoking such as heart disease, cancer and generally poisoning your body. But smoking can also really damage your immune system.

Smoking can do a lot of damage to your lungs, and if your immune system is trying to fight off a respiratory disease (such as the coronavirus) then you are not going to be able to fight it as well as a non smoker will be able to.

Smoking can also reduce the amount of white blood cells that you have which is a vital element of your immune system. With reduced white blood cells, your immune system is in a weaker position to defend you against antigens. In fact, cigarette smoking can stop the production of white blood cells altogether due to the antibodies it can create.

We know that it is not easy to give up smoking, especially if you have been doing it for a long time. But for the sake of your immune system it is essential that you do this. There are plenty of aides around to help you to give up.

Alcohol

This is another thing that you were expecting to be in this chapter wasn't it? People drink for different reasons and in different amounts. The worrying thing is that even the smallest amount of alcohol can lower the amount of white blood cells that you have.

If you drink regularly, or in large quantities, then this is going to damage your immune system. The more that you drink (or the more often), the more you will reduce your white blood cell count and you know how important these are to protect you.

Not only can drinking alcohol reduce your white blood cells, it can also radically change the way that they perform. They can stop trying to fight against antigens, which means that you will be prone to all kinds of diseases and infections.

The good news is that when you stop drinking, your immune system can recover from this and get back to the condition that it needs to be in. Just reducing your alcohol intake can work wonders.

Again giving up drinking is not an easy thing to do. Start off by reducing your intake and go on from there. Remind yourself how important your immune system is the next time someone invites you on an alcoholic binge.

If the coronavirus pandemic is still in force while you are reading this guide, you could find yourself with a lot more time on your hands. This can be stressful, and some people are drinking more to cope with this. Don't do this – put your immune system first.

Leading a Sedentary Lifestyle

These days many people lead too much of a sedentary lifestyle. They travel to work sitting in their car. When they get to their office they sit in front of a computer screen for several hours. Then they travel home sitting in their car and when they arrive home they sit on the couch in front of the TV.

There are two major problems with leading a sedentary lifestyle:

- It can lead to high blood pressure
- It can increase your cholesterol

Your immune system works closely with your heart to form a strong barrier to disease. So it is vital that you do all that you can to keep your heart as healthy as possible.

We realize that in these modern times a lot of people have to work at a job that requires them to sit in front of a computer screen for several hours each day. If you are in this situation then take regular breaks and do some stretches. Daily exercise is very important as well and we will discuss this in a later chapter.

Avoid Stress

This is another thing that is easier said than done, but you must reduce the amount of stress that you experience as much as possible. It is a mistake to think that stress only affects your mental health. Stress can cause a number of physical problems as well.

Stress is another thing that can reduce those all important white blood cells. If you are really stressed then your body produces different hormones faster than usual, and some of these hormones can impair white blood cell production.

If you are a chronic stress sufferer then this is very likely going to increase your blood pressure levels and also negatively impact your digestive system. It is vital that you pay attention to your mental health as well as your physical health to protect your immune system.

There are a variety of techniques available to help you relieve stress. We will discuss relieving stress in more detail in a later chapter. All of the good work that you do to boost your immune system can be totally wiped out if you are always stressed out.

Sleep Deprivation

If you are not getting enough sleep every day then this can have a serious impact on your immune system. When you do not get the right amount of sleep you can find that you get sick more often and it takes a lot longer for you to recover.

When you are asleep your body produces cytokines. These are small proteins that will help the other cells in your immune system to work more effectively. Also during sleep, there are hormones produced that assist your white blood cells to adapt how they fight antigens and deal with them in a more effective way.

If you are struggling to get a good sleep at the moment then creating a consistent schedule will help you. This means going to bed at the same time each night. Your body will get used to this and you will find it easier to fall asleep when the time is right. We will cover sleep in more detail later on.

Don't Eat the wrong Foods

Too many people eat the wrong food these days. There is far too much processed food around now and this can cause inflammation in your body. Our best advice here is to avoid foods that come in cans or boxes because they are likely to have a high salt and sugar content.

If you eat a lot of junk food then you will need to change your diet to one based on whole foods to protect your immune system. Sugary foods should definitely be avoided, as they can damage your metabolism and cause chronic illnesses which will severely weaken your immune system.

- In the next chapter we will discuss immune boosting foods...

Immune System Boosting Foods

The food that you eat is so important for your body and your immune system. You derive most of the antioxidants and nutrients that your body needs from eating the right things. A good diet to boost your immune system and sustain it at high levels will always include the right fruits and vegetables for example.

Your diet needs to provide you with vitamin A, vitamin C, vitamin D, vitamin E and selenium. You are very unlikely to find these in processed foods unless they have been enriched with them. It is far better for you and your immune system to go for whole foods that are fresh.

Some good examples are citrus fruits, nuts and leafy green vegetables. These foods have high levels of the antioxidants and nutrients that you require to give your immune system a great boost. So in this chapter we will specifically point to the best foods for you to consume to bolster your immune system.

Fish

Do you include fish in your diet on a regular basis? If not then you need to change right now. The reason to add fish to your diet is that it contains a great source of selenium. This is particularly true of tuna, which contains the highest levels.

Other types of fish and seafood have selenium in them too and you can mix things up for variety. A great fish to eat to strengthen your immune system is salmon. Salmon has a high degree of omega-3 healthy fat which has been proven to strengthen the immune system and reduce heart disease.

Brazil Nuts

Another great source of selenium can be found in Brazil nuts. You need a good amount of selenium in your diet as it is a powerful antioxidant which is good for an immune system boost. You can get more than the recommended daily amount of selenium through eating a single Brazil nut.

Sunflower Seeds

You should eat sunflower seeds because they contain high levels of vitamin E. An ounce of sunflower seeds can provide you with over 75% of the daily recommended intake of vitamin E. You need vitamin E as it is another powerful antioxidant that bolsters your immune system.

Lentils

A lot of people consume lentils as an alternative to meat or fish but you can include them in any diet. A single cup of lentils will provide a good amount of selenium as well as nutrients to strengthen your immune system and they provide protein and fiber too.

Yogurt

If you eat the right kind of yogurt you will introduce good bacteria (yes there is good bacteria as well as bad) into your body which will fight the bad bacteria and also help with your digestion.

Carrots

Carrots are a delicious vegetable that contain zinc as well as vitamin A, B, C and E. It has been shown many times that zinc is beneficial to our immune systems. In fact if your body is deficient in zinc it will make your immune system weaker.

Garlic

Garlic is another food that provides a good source of zinc. A lot of research has been conducted around garlic with some researchers claiming that it is a good way to keep out the common cold. People suffering with cancer were able to boost their immune system by consuming garlic according to some studies.

Broccoli

You may have heard that broccoli is good for you before and this is true. It contains phytonutrients which can really help to bolster your immune system. One serving of broccoli will provide one third of your daily vitamin A intake and it is also rich in antioxidants.

Spinach

There is a lot of vitamin C in spinach and some vitamin E as well. Keep your spinach raw so that you can get all of the nutrients from it. You can easily add spinach to a sandwich or a salad.

Sweet Potatoes

This is another great tasting vegetable that will provide a good source of vitamin A. Just a single serving of sweet potato will provide over three times your daily recommended intake of vitamin A. It also contains other beneficial antioxidants as well.

Citrus Fruits

You may already be aware that vitamin C is essential for your immune system. Citrus fruits are packed with vitamin C. To get your daily intake just have an orange or a grapefruit for your breakfast and then add some sliced lemon to the water that you drink.

Watermelons

Not everyone is a fan of watermelons but they do contain a lot of nutrients to boost your immune system. Watermelons also contain potassium which is important for the regulation of body functions. It also contains vitamin C and vitamin A.

Blueberries

Did you know that blueberries are full of antioxidants? Well they are – in fact they contain more antioxidants than any other fruit or vegetable. Blueberries are great for strengthening your immune system and they can also help to lower the risk of heart disease, cholesterol and even cancer.

You can get a lot of the nutrients you need from eating pomegranates. They contain a wide variety of antioxidants and they help to fight inflammation as well which is great for your immune system.

Mushrooms

Mushrooms are delicious and they can really help to stimulate your immune system. The Agarikon and Reishi mushrooms have been part of studies that proved they had a beneficial effect on the human immune system.

These studies showed that Reishi mushrooms could interfere with a virus attacking the body and reduce its ability to multiply by attaching to cells. The Agarikon mushroom can be an antibacterial agent and it also has good anti-inflammatory properties.

Turmeric

We close this chapter on immune boosting foods with turmeric. It is a very pleasant spice that you can easily add to your cooking. Turmeric can actually be a poison for cancer cells and it can reduce inflammation as well.

In the next chapter we will discuss supplements to boost your immune system...

Supplements to Bolster Your Immune System

You now know that your immune system is a complex mixture of cells, chemicals and processes that work together to provide you with protection against antigens. It is very important that you do all that you can to boost and maintain your immune system levels so that you can prevent diseases.

We encourage you to follow the advice in the last couple of chapters by avoiding things that can damage your immune system and eating the foods that will boost it. In this chapter we will look at using supplements to provide your immune system with a healthy boost.

While we recommend that you take the advice in this chapter seriously and chose the right supplements, please be aware that the taking of supplements is not guaranteed to prevent diseases and will be very unlikely to cure any diseases that you may currently have.

We will provide you information on supplements here that can bolster your immune system that is based on sound research.

Vitamin D

Vitamin D is one of the most essential nutrients for the proper functioning and overall health of your immune system. It is a fat soluble that increases the fighting abilities of macrophages and monocytes that make up your white blood cells.

Most people just do not get enough vitamin D. When you are deficient in this vitamin it is possible that it can have a negative impact on your immune system. A low level of vitamin D can put you more at risk to respiratory infections like the coronavirus and the flu.

A number of studies showed that using vitamin D supplements can improve the response of the immune system. Some recent research suggested that vitamin D supplements may provide additional protection against respiratory infections.

A review of studies of over 11,000 people in 2019 revealed that using vitamin D supplements significantly lowered the risk of a respiratory infection in people that were deficient, and also lowered the risk of infection in others that had adequate levels of vitamin D.

Vitamin C

A lot of people take vitamin C supplements because they know that is good for their immune system. Vitamin C provides support to immune cell functionality and enhances the ability of these cells to fight off antigens.

Vitamin C also plays an important role in the death of cells. This is vital because the dead cells need clearing out and replacing with new cells so that your immune system can remain healthy. It is also a powerful antioxidant and will help to prevent damage due to oxidative stress.

A big review of a number of case studies involving over 11,000 participants found that by taking vitamin C supplements regularly, adults were able to reduce the duration of the common cold by 8% and children by 14%.

Zinc is a mineral that is critical for the healthy functioning of your immune system. Many supplements contain zinc because it is so vital for the development of immune cells and for the response to inflammation.

You really do not want to be zinc deficient because this could certainly compromise your immune system. But more than 2 billion people across the world have a zinc deficiency and this is especially prevalent in older people.

There have been many studies showing that taking zinc supplements can protect against respiratory infections. It can also help those that are sick already. A study in 2019 of over 60 children in hospital with a respiratory infection found that supplementing zinc intake by a further 30 mg each day reduced their duration of stay by 2 days on average.

Selenium

Being a powerful antioxidant, selenium plays a crucial role in the health of your immune system. It is also an essential mineral for your overall health and wellbeing. As an adult you need to have a daily selenium intake of 55 micrograms per day.

There have been various studies that show viruses thriving in people that are selenium and vitamin E deficient. By taking selenium supplements, there is a good chance that you will provide your immune system with a boost and also minimize inflammation.

The treatment of infections using black elderberry has been practiced for a long time. Various test tube studies revealed that elderberry extract contains potent antiviral and antibacterial properties to fight against pathogens (antigens) which can cause respiratory infections. Studies also showed it to enhance the response of the immune system and reduce severity and duration of colds.

A recent review of four studies with 180 participants found that elderberry supplements reduced upper respiratory symptoms resulting from viral infections significantly. You can obtain elderberry supplements in both capsule and liquid form.

Vitamin E

Like selenium, vitamin E is a strong antioxidant. It will enhance your immune system and help you to fight off disease forming antigens. The experts recommend that you need a 15 mg dose of vitamin E as an adult. If you are deficient in vitamin E then supplements could help.

Medicinal Mushrooms

The use of medicinal mushrooms for the prevention and treatment of disease has been going on since ancient times. There have been studies of a lot of different types of medicinal mushrooms to identify their potential for bolstering the immune system.

These studies concluded that there were more than 270 types of medicinal mushrooms that have the potential to boost the immune system. You may have heard of some of the more commonly known types such as:

- Reishi
- Cordyceps
- Turkey Tail
- Lion's Mane
- Shitake
- Maitake

There was a study conducted with 79 adult participants who were provided with cordyceps mycelium culture supplements. It was discovered that this provided a significant increase of 38% in their natural killer cells, which are a white blood cell type that protects people from infections.

In the next chapter we will discuss ways that you can reduce stress to keep your immune system levels high…

Reducing Stress to Keep Immune System Levels High

Stress is no good for your immune system at all and it can be a significant contributor to the onset of sickness. These days' one in three people claim that they feel very stressed in their life. If this is true then they are at greater risk of becoming sick because the stress will weaken their immune system.

If you feel regularly stressed then you must pay attention to the advice in this chapter. When you are experiencing stress you will lower the ability of your immune system to protect you from harmful antigens. You need to do everything that you can to avoid stress.

By reducing the amount of stress that you experience in your daily life, the stronger your immune system will become. We have a number of suggestions for you and urge you to follow them to reduce the stress in your life. The first of these is all about your diet.

Cut out Coffee and Sugary Beverages

Most people in America and some other westernized countries drink far too much coffee. A lot of people reach for the coffee if they are feeling stressed. But if you introduce too much caffeine into your system then you can suppress your adrenals which will usually make the problem a lot worse.

Introducing a lot of sugar into your body through drinking sodas and other drinks that are sugar laden will not help your stress situation either. If you are stressed (and at other times) it is much better for you to drink healthy warm teas.

Healthy teas can help you to relax and reduce your stress. These restorative teas taste great and will work for you all throughout the day. You can get some great tasting infusions such as lemon and ginger which will help you to combat stress.

Don't Eat White Carbohydrates

What we are talking about here are food products made from refined white flour such as white pasta, processed cereals, and white bread. A lot of these products contain a lot of sugar, salt and other preservatives. These will not help you to reduce your stress.

You are better off eating fresh vegetables and fruits instead to get your carbohydrates. By choosing the right ones (see chapter four) you will get good doses of antioxidants and probiotics that will help to relax you.

Choose the right Protein

When you are suffering from stress it can lead to blood sugar imbalances, and protein provides a stabilizing effect with your blood sugar. When you consume the right proteins you will get a boost in energy and also reduce mood swings, jitteriness and agitation as well as sharpen your brain and improve your sleep.

We have already discussed the benefits of eating fish, but you can add other good protein sources to your diet as well such as:

- Green peas

- Organic chicken
- Tempeh
- Grass fed meat
- Tahini
- Natural yogurt
- Hummus
- Organic eggs
- Quinona
- Seeds
- Nut butters
- Nuts

Making changes to your diet is just one positive thing that you can do to relieve stress. Now we will look at some other great ways to reduce your stress.

Mindfulness Meditation

One of the most powerful ways to relieve stress quickly is to master the art of mindfulness meditation. When you are able to leave all of the stresses of the day behind and focus on the present moment you will find that your stress disappears very quickly.

A lot of people think that mindfulness meditation is a difficult thing to do. They have visions in their head of learning complex yoga poses and sitting in a trance for hours on end. It is not like this at all.

Here is a simple mindfulness meditation practice that you can do right now. You do not require any special equipment such as a bench or couch to do this. Just find a good space and dedicate a little time to the practice.

All you are going to do here is focus your attention on the present moment. When you do this you can leave any judgment behind. If you find your mind wanders then just focus back in the present. It will take a bit of practice but in a short time it will be easy for you.

Use a comfortable and solid seat and pay attention to your legs. Be sure that the bottoms of your feet are resting flat on the floor. Keep your upper body straight without making it stiff. Follow the natural curvature of your spine.

Pay close attention to your breathing. Focus on the actual sensation of breathing and experience the air moving through your mouth or nose as well as the rising and falling of your chest as you breathe.

Develop a Positive Attitude

Positive people are less likely to suffer from sickness and have health problems than negative people according to numerous studies. Optimists tend to have a lot stronger immune systems than pessimists do.

If you are a pessimist then it will take time and consistent effort to transition to having a positive attitude. But it will be worth it as you will reduce your stress levels and help your immune system at the same time.

The way that you react to events in your life is critical. If you see everything in a negative light then this is very likely to induce stress. Conversely, if you have a positive attitude then you will handle situations in life in a much calmer manner.

One of the best ways to transform to a positive attitude is to start practicing gratitude. Think about all of the people and things that you have in your life that you are grateful for. For example, you can be grateful that you are alive, have your family and friends, a roof over your head and food to eat.

Write down three things that you are grateful for each day. Another good way to change to a positive attitude is to write positive affirmations and read these out each day. These statements can be along the lines of "I can do anything that I put my mind to" and "each day I am getting better and better in every way". Try it, they really work.

In the next chapter we will look how exercise and sleep play a crucial role in the health of your immune system...

Exercice and Sleep

There are a lot of research studies that prove there is a link between exercise and a healthy immune system. These studies reveal that exercising on a daily basis can boost your immune system over the course of your life.

One of the other advantages of daily exercising is that it reduces the effects of aging as well. When you get into the habit of exercising regularly you will be setting yourself up for a healthy immune system as you get older. Older people tend to have weaker immune systems, but if you have always exercised regularly then this should not be a problem for you.

Start Simple with Exercise

We wrote this guide during the coronavirus pandemic and depending on where you live there may be some restrictions on you going outside. You need to respect this because flattening the coronavirus curve is essential. If you cannot go outside then you can exercise in your home or out in your yard.

One of the best forms of exercise is walking. Going on a 20 or 30 minute walk each day can do wonders for your immune system. It can be a bit of a challenge doing this at home but you could walk around your yard for a few minutes a day for example.

Something that you can certainly do at home is either Pilates or yoga. There are plenty of videos on YouTube for example, that will show you the basic moves and this is a good place to start. You can move up to more advanced exercise once you have mastered the basics.

Yoga in particular will help you to bolster your immune system. Not only that but it is a great form of exercise as it gets you to really move your body. You can encourage the growth of your T cells by adopting the Cobras pose for a duration of 3 deep breaths.

Once you become more experienced with yoga you can be more adventurous and try the "legs up the wall" pose. This is good because it encourages lymph drainage and increases blood circulation which will help you to relax and reset your nervous system.

Perform Stretches each Day

Your immune system will always perform better when you are in a relaxed state so you can put yourself into this state by performing simple stretching exercises every day. We recommend that you perform a series of stretches for around 10 minutes as soon as you get out of bed every morning.

One stretch that we highly recommend is called the "forward fold". This can really boost your immune system because it forces blood flow into your sinuses which in turn releases any congestion.

There are many different stretches that you can perform that are very easy to do. Look online for ideas to start you off. You certainly do not need to perform stretching for very long to provide the benefit to your immune system. Do two sets of stretches a day in the morning and evening.

Sleep to Boost your Immune System

There are not many things better than getting enough sleep to help your immune system fight off any antigens. It is critical that you get the right amount of sleep as you need to produce the correct levels of cytokines which you can only do while sleeping. This protein helps to reduce infections and inflammation too.

When you get a good sleep every night you will keep your immune system in the best shape to protect you from viruses and bacteria. As an adult you will need between 7 hours and 9 hours of sleep each night so that your body is able to regenerate properly.

We know that sometimes it is not always possible for you to get this amount of sleep each night. If you don't get the sleep that you need then try taking a couple of 30 minute naps during the day to make up for this.

If you have difficulty sleeping then we have some good advice for you to follow. You need to follow this advice because if your body is deprived of sleep then your immune system will not be able to function as it should.

Establish a Routine

It is certainly possible to fool your body into going to sleep at a certain time every day. Do you find that you feel tired at a similar time each day? What you need to do if this is the case is to go to bed just before this time.

You need to setup a routine so that you can do all of the things that you need to do before your designated time to go to bed. If you need to, you can set an alarm to remind you that it is time for you to get ready for bed.

It is not difficult to establish a sleeping time ritual in your life. When you do this you will know that at a specific time each day you can disconnect from all of the day to day stresses and slowly encourage your body that you need to shut down and get some restful sleep.

Preparing for Sleep

You need to create the right atmosphere for sleeping. Take a look at your bedroom and see if it is comfortable enough for you. If your bed is not that comfortable then consider getting a new one that is. Good pillows are essential as well. Falling asleep or staying asleep can be difficult when you are uncomfortable.

What kind of noise levels exist in your bedroom? What temperature is the room? Some people find it helpful to have a constant noise in their bedroom to help them sleep such as a white noise machine or even a simple fan.

Using essential oils on your pillows can also help your brain to relax. We recommend that you switch off any electronics such as a TV in your bedroom, or move it to another room altogether. Having the TV on will not encourage you to sleep as it will stimulate you instead.

Don't drink coffee or anything that contains caffeine at least 3 hours prior to your sleeping time. We recommend that you avoid eating large meals 3 hours before going to bed as well. These things work so be patient and persistent with them. In a short time you will find that you are sleeping well each night.

In the next chapter you will learn how to detoxify your body for a stronger immune system...

Detoxify Your Body for a Stronger Immune System

Your immune system works at its most effective when your body is clean of toxins. The reason for this is that it works a lot less hard when there are no toxins to contend with. The result of this is a stronger fight taking place against antigens that can cause disease.

Detoxifying your body is the practice of cleaning out anything that your cells do not require. This can be a substance that causes harm or something that could prevent your cells from functioning in the correct way. In this chapter we will provide you with six simple methods that you can use to detoxify your body in a natural way.

1. Use Pure Water for Detoxification

One of the best ways to perform a natural body detoxification is to drink pure water. You need to drink quite a lot of water to ensure that you flush out all of the toxins. The key part of this is the "pure water". This means just ordinary water and not carbonated water and certainly no sugary drinks or coffee.

Your body needs water to function properly. So when you provide it with pure water for a period of time it will absorb it easily and then it will eliminate any toxins that are present through bodily fluids such as your sweat and your urine.

2. Drinking Warm Lemon Water to Detoxify

Staying with the water theme, it is a great idea to drink warm lemon water when you wake up each morning. In fact you can drink it anytime during the day. The great thing about warm lemon water is that it is very effective at breaking down those unwanted toxins and assisting your body to eliminate them altogether.

Warm lemon water is a natural diuretic which will clean your urinary tract. It will also provide detoxification for your liver and will give your immune system a much needed boost due to the nutrients that it contains.

3. Eat the right kind of Foods

Eating the right foods has been a common theme throughout this guide and there is very good reason for this. When you consume the right kind of foods you will naturally detoxify your body. So ensure that your diet includes plenty of fresh fruit and vegetables and that you get algae in your diet too.

There are super foods that do a great job in eliminating heavy metals and toxic chemicals from your body. These super foods include:

- Alfalfa
- Blue-green algae
- Cilantro

Another natural and effective way to detox is through fasting. This takes into account how you eat as well as what you eat. So for example you could have a regime where you only consume liquids for a 12 hour or more period, as this will help to significantly reduce your body's toxicity levels.

4. Regular Exercise

You might think that it is strange to see regular exercise as a way to detoxify your body but it does work. The key here is to work up a sweat when you are exercising. Sweating in this way will help you to eliminate toxins a lot more easily. When you sweat after exercise you can get rid of bad toxins such as arsenic, cadmium and mercury for example.

5. Regular Meditation

This is another way of getting a body detox that you might not have thought of. When you meditate you improve the circulation of your blood. You will also boost your metabolism and meditation is great for your cardiovascular system as well.

6. Breathing Clean Air

There is one other great way that you can detoxify your body and that is to get as much fresh, clean air as you can. If the coronavirus pandemic is still in force then this may be difficult to do right now. But when you are able to go outside again chose a destination that has clean air.

You can always improve the air quality in your home and your place of work as well. You can add plants to your environment as these will clean the air. It is very important that you keep your home as dust free as possible.

Make sure that you service your home HVAC system regularly and that this includes cleaning all of the air ducts. It is easy for toxic substances to form in your heating and ventilating system and here are a few examples:

- Microorganisms
- Smoke
- Mold
- Fumes
- Pet hair
- Mildew

If you have a high concentration of these substances in your air ducts (which is pretty likely if you have not cleaned them for a long time) then they can cause your home to become toxic.

So the message here is clear. Eliminate the toxins in your body and your environment so that you can free up your immune system to fight those nasty antigens. It is not difficult to detoxify your body, so do it on a regular basis.

In the next chapter we will discuss the use of essential oils to boost your immune system…

Using Essential Oils to Boost Your Immune System

Did you know that essential oils have been used for hundreds of years for disinfecting and healing? Well they have, and the reason is that an essential oil is an aromatic chemically active compound derived from plants.

Most people think that essential oils are just for pampering. There are products that you add to your bath water, household cleaning products made from essential oils and candles to name but a few.

There has been a great deal of research into essential oils and the conclusion to date is that they have immune boosting characteristics. A lot of people use them in winter when the cold and flu season is at its height and swear that this helps.

The purpose of the essential oils was to protect the plants that they originated from. So it is not too much of a surprise that they can benefit our immune systems as well. A lot of essential oils will bolster your immune system's response to eliminating the antigens and bacteria that cause diseases. Here are some of their immune boosting properties:

- Antiviral
- Anti-inflammatory
- Antibacterial
- Antiseptic
- Antifungal

There are other benefits to using essential oils as well. You can sleep better by using lavender essential oil. To relieve anxiety and stress you can use jasmine. Here are the best essential oils that you should use to boost your immune system:

1. Frankincense

You probably heard about this at school when you were learning about the birth of Jesus and the three wise men bearing gifts. Frankincense is an extract from the Boswellia tree which is well known across the world for its anti-inflammatory properties.

Frankincense is able to fight inflammation due to four acids from the tree that help your many inflammatory pathways. The most powerful of these acids is AKBA (acetyl-11-keto-β-boswellic acid).

Different scientific studies have discovered a direct link between the ability of frankincense to reduce inflammation and a stronger immune system. When you use it topically, frankincense will give your immune system a boost and reduce inflammation. It also provides faster healing and tissue remodeling.

Frankincense also contains strong antioxidants to quell free radicals and protects your immune system from a poor diet, industrial toxins and environmental pollutants. It is an amazing essential oil.

2. Eucalyptus

Eucalyptus has been used for a very long time as a decongestant and is found in a lot of cold and flu remedies. It contains a compound called 1,8-cineole which has strong antioxidant, anti-inflammatory and antibacterial properties.

In a study that was published in the Clinical Microbiology and Infection journal, it was discovered that eucalyptus provided different antibacterial effects on a number of infectious bacteria in the respiratory tract. This included strains that caused strep.

Other studies reported that merely inhaling eucalyptus fights bacteria that cause Staphylococcus aureus and tuberculosis. Eucalyptus can also stimulate your innate immune system by enhancing the phagocytic responsiveness to pathogens.

3. Oregano

You have probably heard of oregano before because it is widely used in Mexican and Italian cooking. But it also has powerful antibacterial characteristics due to the high levels of two active compounds it contains which are thymol and carvacrol. These will kill bacterial cells because they make the membranes more permeable.

Harmful bacteria are compromised when this happens and they will leak critical molecules for their survival. Tests have shown oregano oil killing E. coli, Salmonella and a number of Staphylococcus bug types.

In a 2017 study, it was found that oregano essential oil has very good antioxidant properties as well which help to boost the immune system. Oregano will also inhibit several viruses including norovirus, anti-biotic resistant herpes, a number of respiratory viruses and the rotavirus.

4. Thyme

Thyme is rich in thymol like oregano is. This can help to reduce coughing symptoms that are associated with a number of respiratory infections. A study combined thyme with ivy and found that this reduced more than 68% of coughing fits among people that had acute bronchitis.

But thyme does more than just relieve symptoms. Thyme essential oil produces a high level of non specific immune and antimicrobial activity. Studies have shown it to be effective against a range of bacteria, including treatment resistant strains such as MRSA.

Use the Power of Essential Oils to Boost your Immune System

We have highlighted the best four essential oils for boosting your immune system in this chapter. They can help to bolster your immune system both directly and indirectly. So we strongly recommend that you make essential oils part of your everyday life so that you can strengthen your immune system.

In the final chapter we will show you the best practices that you need to follow to boost your immune system...

Best Practices to Boost Your Immune System

We have a number of best practices that we strongly encourage you to follow to boost your immune system. These are all proven ways that you can develop the strongest possible immune system that will provide you with the maximum protection against disease.

1. Understand the Benefits of a Strong Immune System

To make the necessary lifestyle changes that will result in a healthy immune system it is essential that you understand the benefits that this will bring to you. Your immune system is vital for protecting you from disease and it is very precious so you need to do everything that you can to keep it strong.

2. Know what your Immune System does and how it works

By knowing what your immune system does and how it works to protect you is important because it will motivate you to make the changes in your life that you know will make it stronger. Some of these changes will not be easy for you but they will be worth it.

You do not need to be a doctor to understand how it works – just be aware of the innate and adaptive immune systems as well as the role of your lymphatic system and how these all work together to protect you.

3. Avoid the things known to compromise your Immune System

There are some things that you may be doing at the moment that will compromise your immune system and make it weaker. You want to avoid activities such as smoking and drinking alcohol to excess as these will damage your immune system over time.

Avoiding stress will certainly help to protect your immune system. These days most people are leading a sedentary lifestyle and this can harm your immune system as well. Eating the wrong foods and depriving yourself of the correct amount of sleep are also things to avoid.

4. Eat Foods that Boost your Immune System

The food that you consume is vital for the state of your immune system. Your food provides you with the nutrients and antioxidants that your immune system needs to stay strong. Changing to a diet that has a high fruit and vegetable count is the right thing to do.

Your diet needs to provide you with the right amount of vitamins C, D and E as well as selenium. These essential vitamins are not present in processed foods so eliminate these from your diet. We understand that changing your diet is a big step to take, but you must do it for the sake of your immune system.

5. Take Immune System Boosting Supplements

There are a variety of supplements available today that will help to strengthen your immune system. Look for supplements that are rich in the essential vitamins C, D and E as well as zinc and selenium. Black elderberry is something that you should look at and so are medicinal mushrooms such as reishi and cordyceps.

There is a great deal of evidence around that proves stress is bad for your immune system. You cannot completely eliminate stress but you can do a lot to reduce it. A simple thing to do is to reduce the amount of caffeine, sugar and white carbohydrates you consume.

Mindfulness meditation is a great way to reduce stress because it forces you to live in the moment. It is not difficult to do and very effective. You can also take steps to develop a more positive outlook in your life as negativity will increase stress.

7. Exercise and Sleep well

Regular exercise is a great way to maintain a healthy immune system. If you are not exercising regularly right now then you can start in a gentle way and gradually do more. Change your routine to get the right amount of sleep every night. You can establish a new schedule and trick your body into wanting to sleep at the same time each day.

8. Detoxify your body

When your body is clear of toxins your immune system will be a lot more effective. This is because it can focus on detecting harmful pathogens and not have to contend with toxins as well. There are a number of methods that you can use to detoxify your body such as drinking pure water, eating healthily and breathing clean air.

9. Use Essential Oils to boost your Immune System

Essential oils are not just there so that you can pamper yourself. Some of them contain characteristics that will help to boost your immune system such as antiviral, anti-inflammatory, antibacterial, antiseptic and antifungal properties. The top essential oils are frankincense, eucalyptus, oregano and thyme.

Conclusion

You now know what your immune system does, how it works and what you can do to boost it and maintain it in its optimum state. There are a lot of things that you can do to strengthen your immune system and we recommend that you create a plan to introduce these into your life.

Now more than ever, it is essential that you take good care of your immune system and do all that you can to bolster it. With the coronavirus pandemic and other threats to your health, having a strong immune system will go a long way to protecting you and preventing you from becoming sick.

So we urge you to take these immune boosting tips seriously and start to use them today.

If you enjoyed this book, please let me know your thoughts by leaving a short review on Amazon.

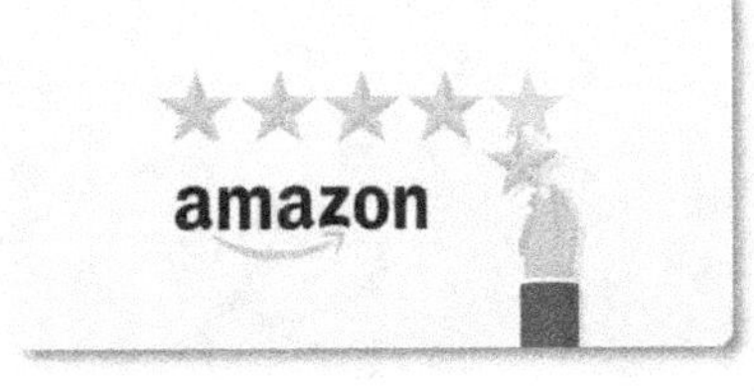

Thank you!